HOW YOUR IMMUNE SYSTEM WORKS

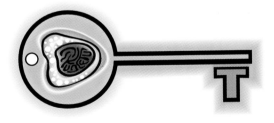

HOW YOUR IMMUNE SYSTEM WORKS DESCRIBES THE IMMUNE SYSTEM IN GENERAL AND DISCUSSES MANY COMMON CONDITIONS AND DISORDERS. IT TRIES TO MAKE YOU A SMARTER CONSUMER OF HEALTH SERVICES AND PRODUCTS, BUT IT DOES NOT OFFER MEDICAL ADVICE AND IS NOT A SUBSTITUTE FOR MEDICAL CARE OR SUPERVISION. CONSULT A PHYSICIAN ABOUT ALL YOUR SPECIFIC HEALTH CONCERNS.

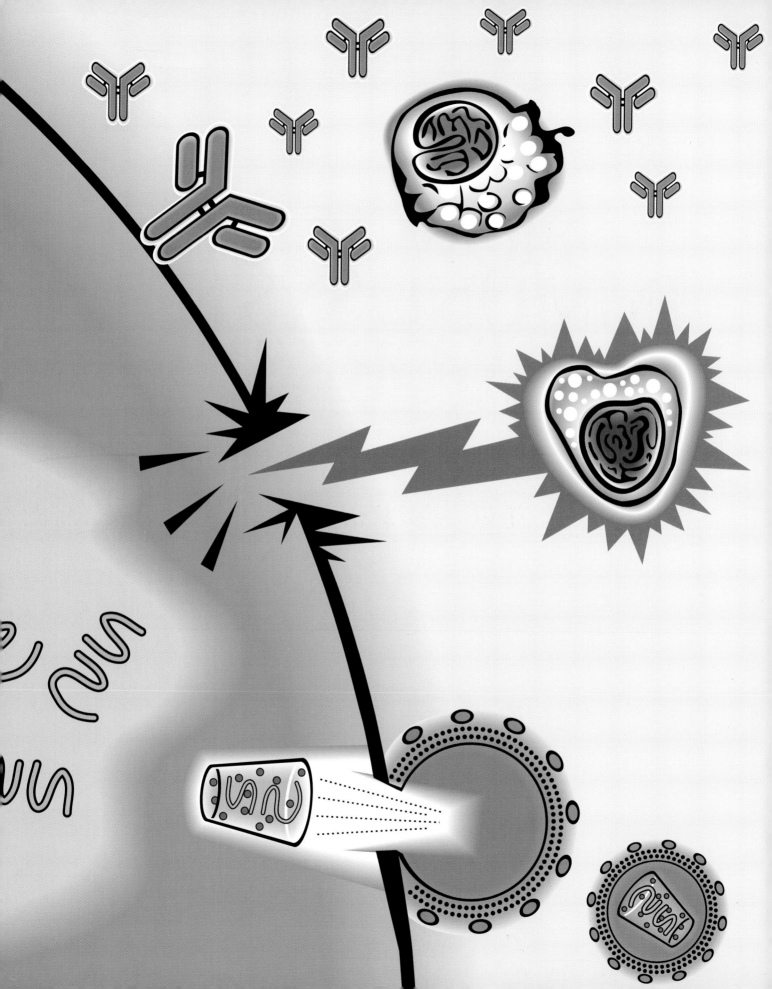

HOW YOUR IMMUNE SYSTEM WORKS

JEFF BAGGISH, M.D.

Illustrated by
SCOTT MACNEILL

Ziff-Davis Press
Emeryville, California

Editor	Carol Vartanian
Technical Reviewer	Donna Curtis
Project Coordinator	Ami Knox
Proofreader	Ami Knox
Cover Illustration	Scott MacNeill
Cover Design	Regan Honda
Book Design	Carrie English
Technical Illustration	Scott MacNeill
Word Processing	Howard Blechman
Page Layout	Bruce Lundquist
Indexer	Jeff Baggish, M.D.

Ziff-Davis Press books are produced on a Macintosh computer system with the following applications: FrameMaker®, Microsoft® Word, QuarkXPress®, Adobe Illustrator®, Adobe Photoshop®, Adobe Streamline™, MacLink®*Plus*, Aldus® FreeHand™, Collage Plus™.

If you have comments or questions or would like to receive a free catalog, call or write:
Ziff-Davis Press
5903 Christie Avenue
Emeryville, CA 94608
1-800-688-0448

ISBN 1-56276-233-8

Manufactured in the United States of America
✪ This book is printed on paper that contains 50% total recycled fiber of which 20% is de-inked postconsumer fiber.
10 9 8 7 6 5 4 3 2 1

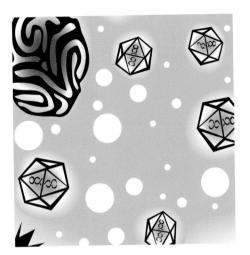

This book is dedicated to my loving wife, Doneene, who stuck with me through years of indecision until I finally found my niche.

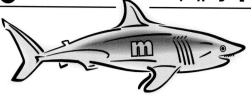

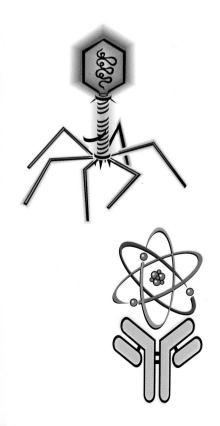

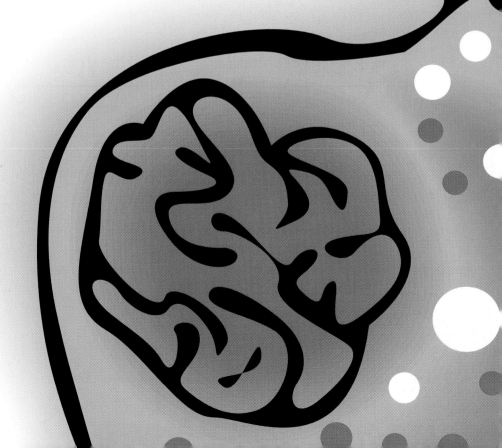

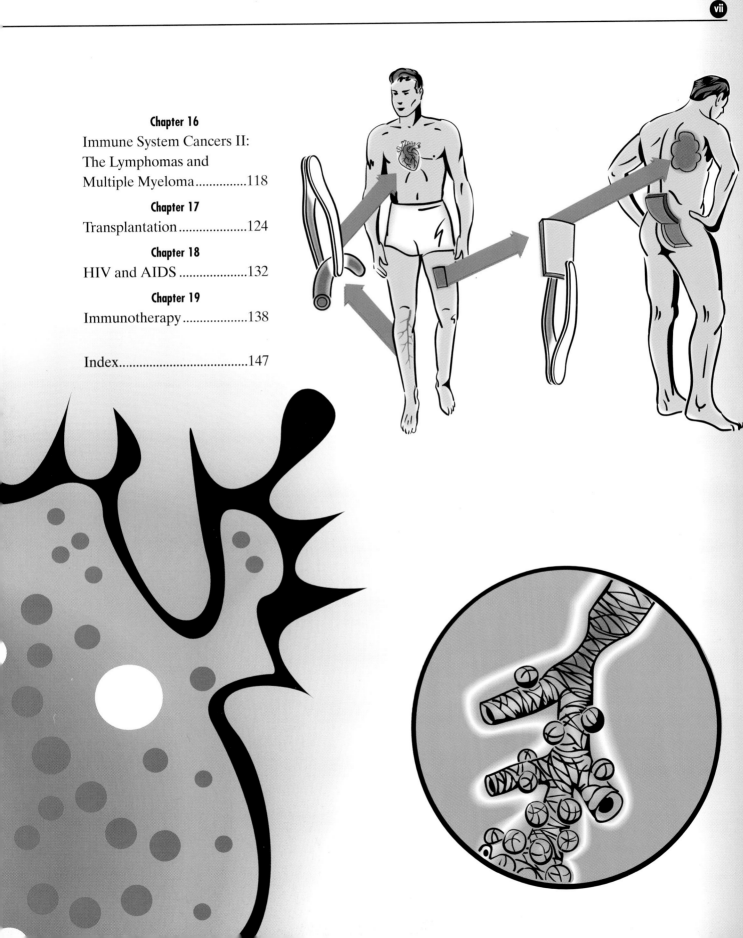

Writing this book would have been impossible were it not for the invaluable contributions of many intelligent and hardworking people. In particular, I wish to thank Eric Stone, Carol Vartanian, Scott MacNeill, Cindy Hudson, Ami Knox, Donna Curtis, Cheryl Holzaepfel, Howard Blechman, Bruce Lundquist, Elisabeth Beller, Margaret Hill, and all the folks at Ziff-Davis Press.

When I would tell people that I was writing a book about the immune system, their reaction was invariably, "Oh, you're writing a book about AIDS?" This is a natural response. I imagine that few people would have been interested in a book about the immune system before AIDS worked its way into the public consciousness. Today, however, most people are at least aware of the immune system, if not intrigued by it. So, my answer to their question is, yes, I have written a book about AIDS—and much more!

Immunology, which is the study of the immune system, is a vast scientific field that includes all of the cells, chemicals, and organs that defend the body against disease. Everything from white blood cells to allergies, from bone marrow to lymph nodes, from vaccines to transplant rejection, and from leukemia to AIDS falls under the heading of immunology. It is a very complex subject, but I have always believed that it would be a source of great fascination for people from all walks of life, if only someone would make it easy to understand. Thus, it has been my objective, through a unique combination of text and illustrations, to make your journey into the world of the immune system both educational and enjoyable.

I have tried to arrange the chapters in a logical sequence, so that you can gradually acclimate yourself to the subject matter rather than be inundated with a flood of technical information all at once. The first five chapters deal strictly with the basics—the cast of immune system characters and their individual roles. Then, armed with a general understanding of what makes up the immune system, you may proceed to the next five chapters, which explain the day-to-day functioning of the various immune system components. After completing ten chapters, you should know more about how the immune system behaves under normal circumstances than you ever thought you could!

Chapters 11 to 18 deal with the problems that arise when the immune system doesn't function ideally. Beginning with allergies, which are the most common immune system–related problem, you will continue on through autoimmune diseases, immune system cancers, transplant rejection, and finally AIDS. By this time, you will be familiar with all the common diseases of the immune system, and you will be ready to take on the final chapter, which deals with the many ways in which the immune system can be manipulated in order to treat illnesses.

I would never presume to offer this book as the final authority on the subject of immunology. My editors and I continually debated about what should be added, deleted, or changed until the very moment the manuscript went to press. After reading the book, you may decide that certain important issues were covered inadequately or not at all. Therefore, I welcome any comments or criticism that might help in the preparation of future editions. Finally, keep in mind that this book should be used as an educational tool only and not as a source for medical advice. No book is a substitute for a visit to your doctor's office.

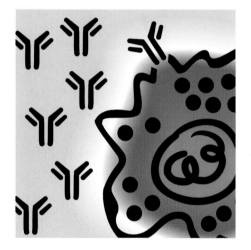

CHAPTER

What Is the Immune System?

OUR BODIES ARE continuously under attack from a sweeping variety of toxins, germs, and pollutants. We breathe air that is saturated with smoke, carbon monoxide, dirt particles, fumes, and chemicals. We handle waste products, garbage, and objects whose travel history we'd rather not know. Cancer cells repeatedly arise in various organs, determined to multiply until they've taken control of the whole body. We eat food teeming with bacteria and drink water that, under a microscope, looks more like a biology experiment than a refreshment. In fact, for 24 hours a day, 7 days a week, from the moment we're born until the moment we die, we endure a continuous barrage from countless enemies who want to control us for their own gain.

It is a wonder that we survive, much less remain reasonably healthy for most of our lives. When we do get sick, we usually manage to heal ourselves in a relatively short time. How is it that we can win battle after battle when the opposition seems to have every advantage? The answer lies in our remarkable means of defense, *the immune system*.

The immune system is an amazingly intricate collection of specialized and not-so-specialized cells, organs, and structures, the mission of which is to identify and destroy foreign invaders before harm is done to the body. Disease-causing organisms, such as bacteria, viruses, fungi, and parasites, are detected upon entry, tagged for termination, and devoured by hungry immune system cells. Cancer cells are similarly recognized as not being welcome and are eliminated. Transplanted organs, although used for lifesaving purposes, are actually foreign objects and are regarded as such by the immune system. Medical science has devoted considerable effort to preventing rejection of transplants.

In fact, the immune system is so aggressive in attacking enemies, that it sometimes overshoots the mark and becomes *too* aggressive. An allergic reaction is an excessive response to a relatively benign intruder, such as pollen, grass, or dust. Even worse, the immune system may mistake a normal body structure or organ for a foreign intruder and attack it, thus causing an autoimmune disease.

Most of us enjoy the protection of a normally functioning immune system, and we take it for granted. However, the alternative can be devastating. In diseases such as cancers of the immune system, like leukemia, lymphoma, and multiple myeloma, abnormal cells run amuck, causing severe illness and often death. The AIDS epidemic has brought new attention to the consequences wrought by a malfunctioning immune system.

Humankind has long been fascinated by the immune system and has sought not only to understand how it works but also to harness its power to treat disease. Vaccines are now routinely given to prevent diseases that were once widespread; smallpox has been virtually eradicated from the planet, and, if immunization programs achieve their goal, polio could soon follow. Modern medical technology increasingly allows us to utilize various components of the immune system in treating once-untreatable diseases.

It may seem futile for anyone but the most accomplished scientists to deal with such a complex subject. This aura of overwhelming complexity prevents many people from even *trying* to understand it. However, when broken down into basic elements and described in plain English, the immune system is not only understandable but fascinating.

Targets of the Immune System

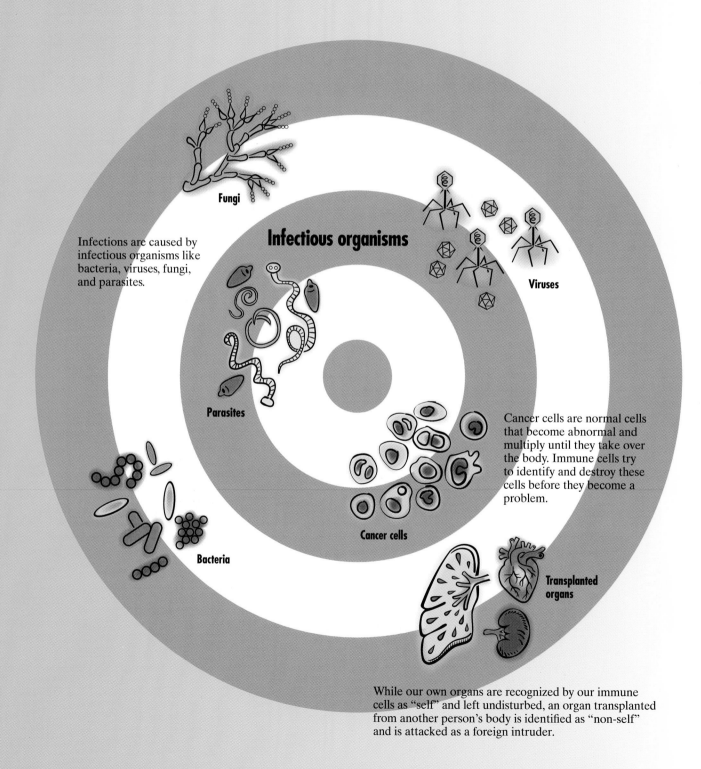

Fungi

Infectious organisms

Viruses

Infections are caused by infectious organisms like bacteria, viruses, fungi, and parasites.

Parasites

Cancer cells are normal cells that become abnormal and multiply until they take over the body. Immune cells try to identify and destroy these cells before they become a problem.

Bacteria

Cancer cells

Transplanted organs

While our own organs are recognized by our immune cells as "self" and left undisturbed, an organ transplanted from another person's body is identified as "non-self" and is attacked as a foreign intruder.

The Immune System's Cast of Characters

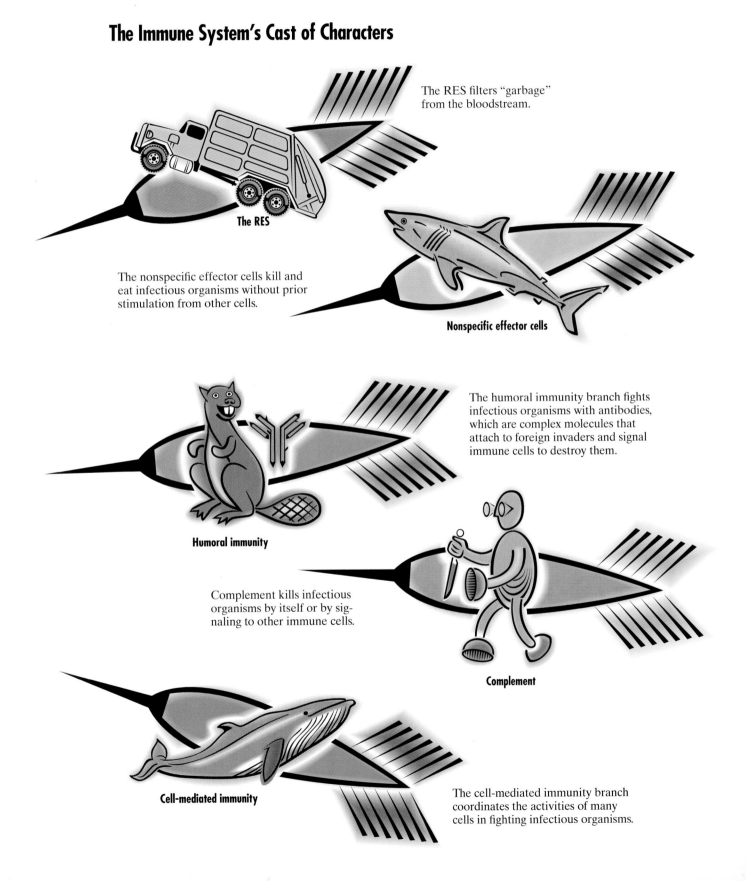

The RES filters "garbage" from the bloodstream.

The RES

The nonspecific effector cells kill and eat infectious organisms without prior stimulation from other cells.

Nonspecific effector cells

The humoral immunity branch fights infectious organisms with antibodies, which are complex molecules that attach to foreign invaders and signal immune cells to destroy them.

Humoral immunity

Complement kills infectious organisms by itself or by signaling to other immune cells.

Complement

Cell-mediated immunity

The cell-mediated immunity branch coordinates the activities of many cells in fighting infectious organisms.

How Allergies Occur

Any substance that irritates the immune system into creating an allergic reaction is called an allergen. Allergens exist in many varieties, and allergy sufferers are affected by them in many different ways.

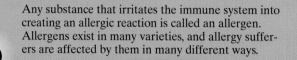

Insect stings

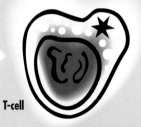

Macrophage

When an allergen invades the body, it is eaten by an immune cell called the macrophage, which presents it to another immune cell, the T-cell.

T-cell

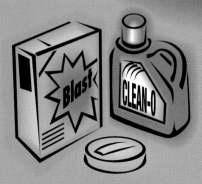

Soaps and detergents

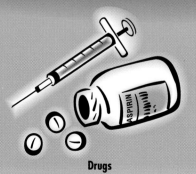

Drugs

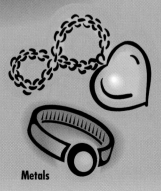

Metals

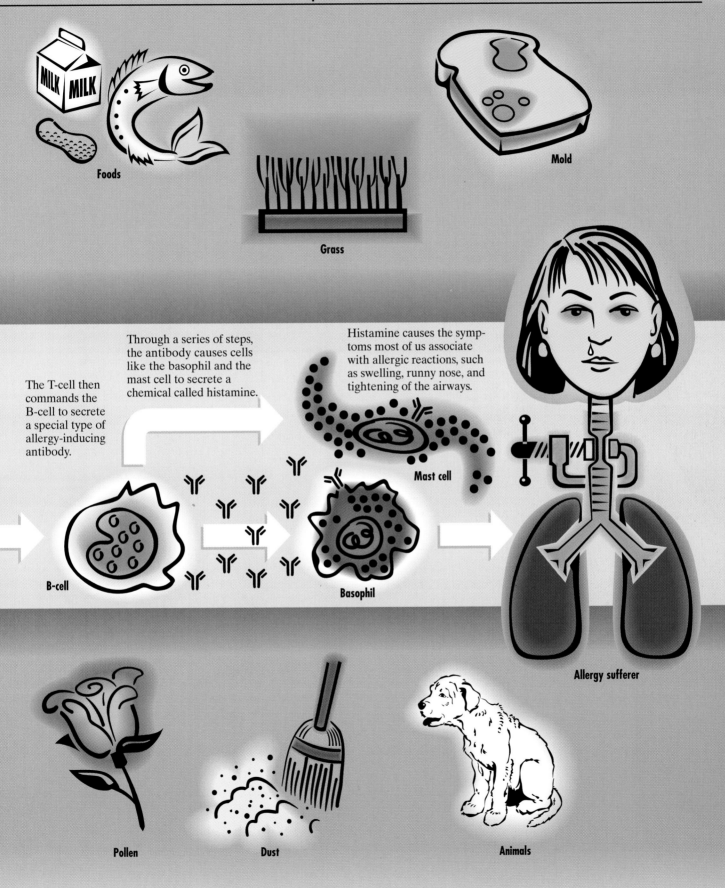

Foods

Grass

Mold

The T-cell then commands the B-cell to secrete a special type of allergy-inducing antibody.

Through a series of steps, the antibody causes cells like the basophil and the mast cell to secrete a chemical called histamine.

Histamine causes the symptoms most of us associate with allergic reactions, such as swelling, runny nose, and tightening of the airways.

Mast cell

B-cell

Basophil

Allergy sufferer

Pollen

Dust

Animals

Immune System Diseases and Immunotherapy

Organs Affected by Autoimmune Diseases

When the immune system mistakes normal "self" organs for foreign "non-self" organs, autoimmune diseases result.

Brain and spinal cord
In multiple sclerosis, immune cells attack the sheath surrounding the spinal cord and brain, causing numbness, tingling, weakness, visual impairment, loss of coordination, and other disturbances.

Thyroid gland
In Graves' disease, immune cells stimulate the thyroid gland to secrete excessive amounts of thyroid hormone, causing bulging eyes, goiter, thickening of skin in the legs, nervousness, increased heart rate, sweating, fatigue, and weight loss.

Skin, Heart, Lungs, and Kidneys
Lupus can cause many different symptoms in multiple organs, including skin rashes, heart and lung inflammation, and kidney damage.

Pancreas
Immune cells attacking the insulin-producing cells of the pancreas is one suspected cause of diabetes. When insulin production disappears, so does the body's ability to control the level of sugar in the blood.

Joint
Joint linings are targeted in rheumatoid arthritis, leading to the pain and disability associated with this disease.

Immune System Malignancies

Leukemia
In leukemia, abnormal white blood cells rapidly multiply at the expense of normal immune function.

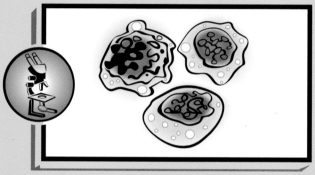

Lymphoma
Lymphoma is an abnormal multiplication of cells in the RES, the body's filtration and garbage disposal system.

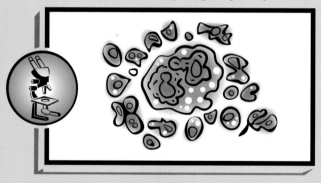

Multiple myeloma
Antibody-producing plasma cells proliferate out of control in multiple myeloma.

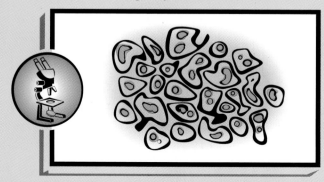

Immunotherapy

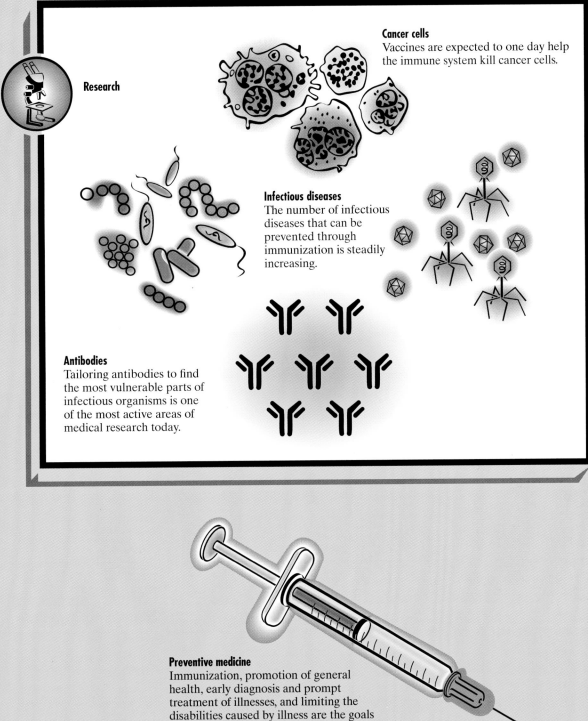

Research

Cancer cells
Vaccines are expected to one day help the immune system kill cancer cells.

Infectious diseases
The number of infectious diseases that can be prevented through immunization is steadily increasing.

Antibodies
Tailoring antibodies to find the most vulnerable parts of infectious organisms is one of the most active areas of medical research today.

Preventive medicine
Immunization, promotion of general health, early diagnosis and prompt treatment of illnesses, and limiting the disabilities caused by illness are the goals of preventive medicine.

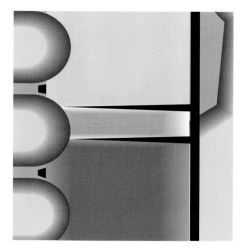

Components of Your Immune System

YOU CAN THINK of the immune system as the body's own defense department, with several branches. Each branch serves a specific purpose and also works in conjunction with the others to achieve a common goal: protecting the body against foreign invasion.

White blood cells are the backbone of the immune system. If you've ever cut yourself and taken a good look at your blood, you may have thought of it as a red, homogeneous liquid. But if you place some of your blood in a test tube and allow it to stand for a while, it will separate into different components. Spinning the tube in a centrifuge will cause separation into even more distinct layers. At the bottom, taking up about half the space, is a layer of *red blood cells*. These cells give the blood its red color and are responsible for carrying oxygen to the far reaches of the body. Occupying the top half is a layer of clear, yellow fluid called *serum*. This is the fluid in which the blood cells are suspended as they course through the body; without it, the blood would be too thick to flow freely. The white blood cells in the test tube are confined to a thin layer sandwiched between the red cells and the serum, called the *buffy coat*. Red cells outnumber white cells by half-a-million to one, but for what white cells lack in numbers, they compensate in sheer ability.

There are many types of white blood cells, and they perform a wide variety of functions, as we shall discuss in Chapters 4 and 5. For now, we can divide the white blood cells into three broad categories with respect to their roles in immune function. The first is the *humoral immunity* component. These specialized white blood cells, called *B-cells,* secrete *antibodies* to fight off foreign invaders. The second branch is the *cell-mediated immunity*, which includes specialized white blood cells, called *T-cells*, that coordinate the activities of multiple segments of the immune system in mounting an efficient attack against the enemy. The third category consists of *nonspecific effector cells*. Unlike the cells of the first two groups, these white blood cells do not have a specialized function and can kill and eat intruders without outside assistance.

Certain white blood cells also play important roles in the *reticuloendothelial system,* or *RES.* The RES comprises immune system cells in the spleen, lymph nodes, liver, bone marrow, lungs, and intestines. It, along with the *lymphatic system*, is the body's sanitation department and is responsible for disposing of the "garbage" that pollutes the blood. RES structures also serve as sites where immune cells wait until foreign invasion triggers their activation. The RES and the lymphatic system will be discussed in greater detail in Chapter 10.

While cells of the humoral and cell-mediated immunity branches must undergo a time-consuming selection process that ensures that each cell will recognize only a specific foreign invader, another immune system branch, the *complement system*, has the ability to identify and destroy enemies on first sight. Complement is a substance that can not only bind to trespassing cells and bacteria for the purpose of attracting other immune cells that can eat the invaders, but it also can kill invading organisms outright by poking holes in their "skin" and allowing in a flood of water. More information on complement appears in Chapter 6.

Many other nonspecific defense mechanisms are at the body's disposal. Mucus is secreted throughout the body and can trap and kill alien material. The stomach produces acid that is so strong that it can kill most toxins or germs we might swallow. Friendly bacteria live in the intestinal tract and stave off attacks from unwelcome visitors. Hairs in our noses and ears keep out particles of dust and dirt; tears and saliva serve similar functions in the eyes and mouth, respectively. A unique apparatus of mucus and microscopic hairs called the *mucociliary blanket* or *elevator* catches pollutants in the air we breathe before they reach the lungs, and carries them upward to where they can be coughed out or swallowed.

The human body's defense mechanism is multifaceted. Each branch has a different assigned task, but their jurisdictions overlap. One component helps another, one picks up where another leaves off, one acts as gatekeeper or filter to another's backup role, and so on. It is a tremendously complex machine that depends on the smooth functioning of all parts. But there would be no reason for this machine to exist at all, were it not for the enemies that would wage war against our bodies. In Chapter 3, we will familiarize ourselves with these enemies, then in later chapters, we will disassemble the immune system into its individual parts in order to understand how it works as a whole.

Blood Composition

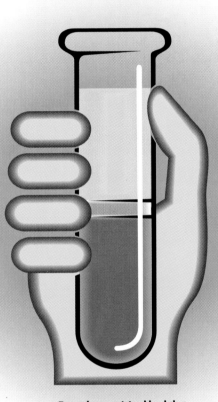

Blood cells float in this clear, straw-colored fluid called serum.

White blood cells, also called leukocytes, are found in this thin layer known as the buffy coat.

Red blood cells, also called erythrocytes, are denser than white cells or serum and, therefore, sink to the bottom.

Test tube containing blood that has been centrifuged to show its components.

Branches of the Immune System

White blood cells, also called leukocytes, are the backbone of the immune system and are grouped into the humoral, cell-mediated, and nonspecific effector cell branches.

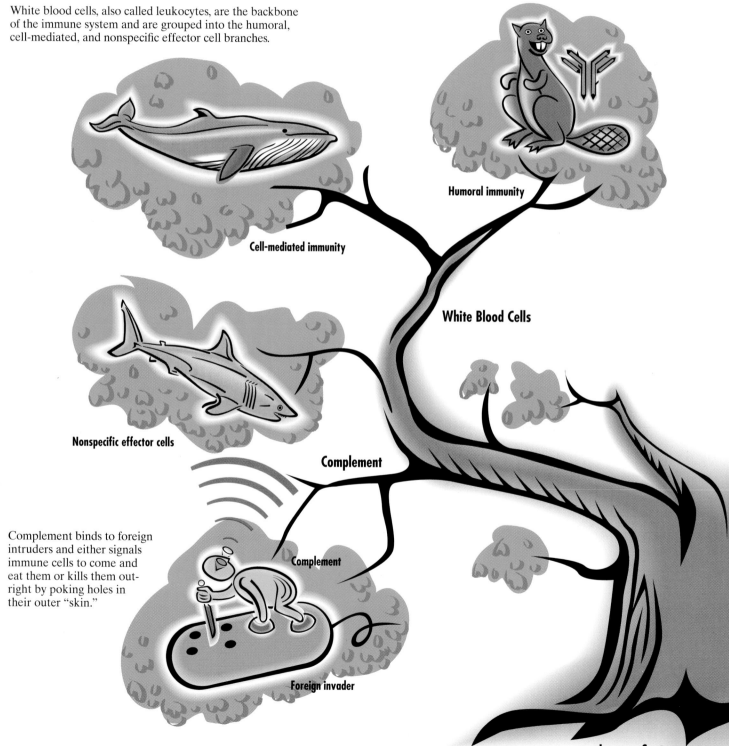

Humoral immunity

Cell-mediated immunity

White Blood Cells

Nonspecific effector cells

Complement

Complement binds to foreign intruders and either signals immune cells to come and eat them or kills them outright by poking holes in their outer "skin."

Complement

Foreign invader

Immune System

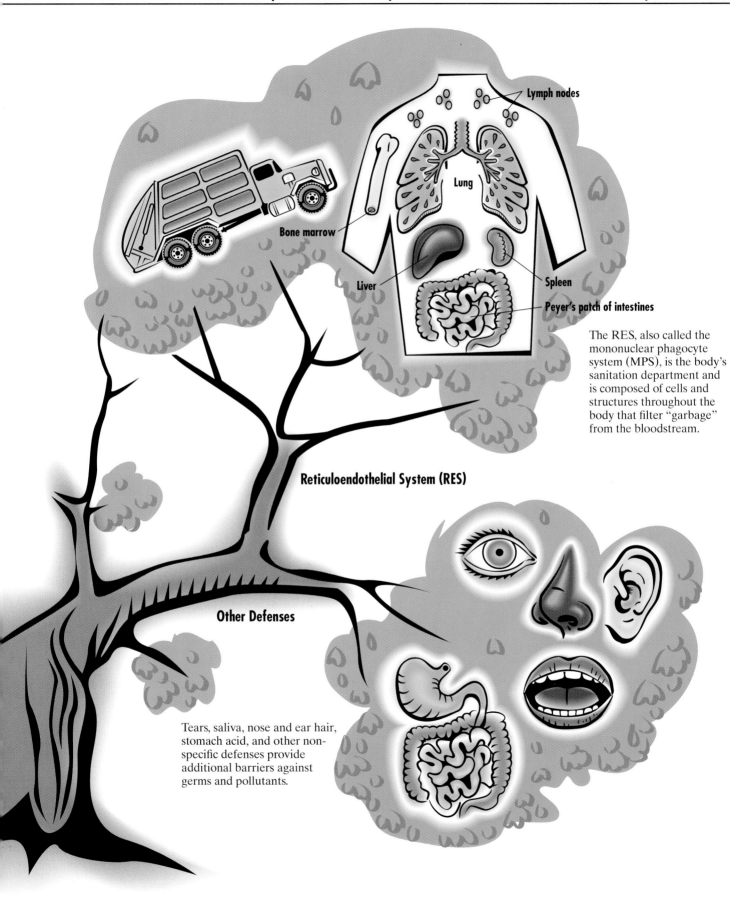

Lymph nodes

Lung

Bone marrow

Liver

Spleen

Peyer's patch of intestines

The RES, also called the mononuclear phagocyte system (MPS), is the body's sanitation department and is composed of cells and structures throughout the body that filter "garbage" from the bloodstream.

Reticuloendothelial System (RES)

Other Defenses

Tears, saliva, nose and ear hair, stomach acid, and other non-specific defenses provide additional barriers against germs and pollutants.

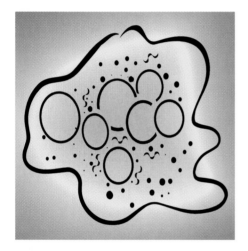

CHAPTER 3

Your Immune System's Enemies

T HAS BEEN said that one should keep a keener eye on one's enemies than on one's friends. This wisdom also applies to anyone seeking to understand the immune system. All its elaborateness would be irrelevant if there were no prey on which to set its sights. For this reason, we will begin our journey by acquainting ourselves with the immune system's most common targets.

People typically think of the immune system as a means of fighting off infection. Though not its sole function, it clearly is its most important one. What exactly is meant by infection? Simply put, an *infection* is an invasion of a particular part of the body by an *infectious organism*. What, then, is an infectious organism?

There are basically four types of infectious organism: bacteria, viruses, fungi, and parasites. Any of these are capable of entering the body, multiplying, and causing an infection. Some infectious organisms, such as those that cause tuberculosis, syphilis, "walking" pneumonia, and Rocky Mountain spotted fever, do not fall neatly into any one class, but they generally are assigned to the bacteria category. Let's examine each group individually.

The *bacterium* is the smallest living organism that can eat, grow, and multiply on its own. Seen even under the highest power of a typical microscope, they are still very small. Some are round like little balls and are called *cocci*. Others are shaped like little hot dogs and are called *bacilli* or *rods*. Some cocci travel in pairs, chains, or clusters. Some bacilli are stretched out long and thin or are wavy. Some bacteria have little tails that help them swim. Others have little hairs or fingers that help them attach to various surfaces. Some are surrounded by protective capsules, others are not. Some breathe oxygen, others don't.

However, all bacteria have certain things in common. All contain the necessary ingredients for eating, generating energy, and reproducing, tucked neatly inside a thin lining, or *membrane*, that is protected by a *cell wall*. All can cause infection of various organs of the body, along with the illness, fever, and pus production that usually accompany it. Although the immune system is adept at fighting off bacterial infections, sometimes it is overwhelmed. Before the development of sulfa drugs and penicillin in the 1930s and '40s, people often died from bacterial infections. Today, however, antibiotics are so effective in treating bacterial infections, that such catastrophes are rare.

A *virus* is a completely different type of infectious organism. Besides being much smaller than a bacterium, it is not self-sufficient and depends on invading a living cell and using the cell's own machinery in order to reproduce. Some viruses, in fact, specialize in injecting themselves into bacteria in order to multiply. The *virion* itself (one virus particle) is extremely simple. All it comprises is a piece of genetic material, such as *DNA* or *RNA*, surrounded by an icosahedral, helical, or complex-shaped shell. DNA stands for *deoxyribonucleic acid*, an extremely complex molecule found inside every cell of the body and responsible for making us and all cellular organisms the way we are. It is the code that determines everything from the color of our hair to the shape of our earlobes. RNA stands for *ribonucleic acid* and is similar to DNA but simpler.

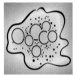

Once inside a living cell, a virus claims the cell as its own and uses it to multiply. New virions scatter to invade other cells, and the infection spreads. To make matters worse, the antibiotics that are so effective against bacteria are completely useless against viruses. Antiviral agents are available to combat a few select viruses, but treatment for the more serious viruses, such as polio, hepatitis B, and measles, centers mostly on prevention through vaccination. Fortunately, the immune system does a great job at fighting off most of the many viral illnesses we suffer in a lifetime.

Everyone is familiar with molds, mushrooms, and yeasts. These are examples of *fungi*. You can think of fungi as life-forms that are slightly more advanced than bacteria but not as advanced as plants. Only a few of the many thousands of fungi create problems for humans. Even when they do, the conditions are usually minor, such as ringworm, athlete's foot, yeast infections, and diaper rash.

On rare occasions, however, fungal infections can be deadly. Certain fungi are classified as *opportunistic organisms* that spread by taking advantage of the weakened immune system of a person with diabetes or AIDS, for example, or of a person who is being treated with immunosuppressant drugs. One such fungus, which is seen occasionally in diabetic individuals, can literally consume a person's face and brain in a matter of days, leading to blindness, coma, and death; only emergency surgery to remove all the diseased tissue is helpful. The brain and spinal cord of people with AIDS often become infected with opportunistic fungi as well. These examples demonstrate how devastating a compromised immune system can be.

Parasites are organisms that grow, feed, and are sheltered on or within other organisms, while contributing nothing in return. They range in size from the microscopic amœba to tapeworms over 30 feet in length. The majority of parasitic diseases, such as malaria and schistosomiasis, occur in developing countries and are contracted by eating contaminated or poorly cooked food. Most can be cured with an appropriate antiparasitic agent.

In addition to targeting infectious organisms, the immune system battles cancer cells as well. *Cancer* occurs when a cell in a body organ becomes abnormal, multiplies uncontrollably, and takes over the entire organ or even the entire body. The immune system is effective at identifying and destroying abnormal cells, especially those made abnormal by a virus or carcinogen, before they become a problem. Sometimes, however, cancer spreads too quickly for the immune system to catch up, and many people ultimately succumb to the disease despite numerous advances in cancer treatment.

Finally, there are many agents that cause allergies. An *allergy* is an overreaction of a person's immune system to a harmless foreign substance. These substances, called *allergens*, include pollen, grasses, molds, dust, insect stings, animal hair, certain foods and drugs, and so on. Though they are not enemies in the same sense as infectious organisms and cancer cells, they cause serious problems for allergy sufferers. Allergies will be discussed in greater detail in Chapters 11 and 12.

Infectious Organisms

Bacteria

Bacteria are the smallest independent living organisms. They exhibit many different features that allow them to adapt to specific environments.

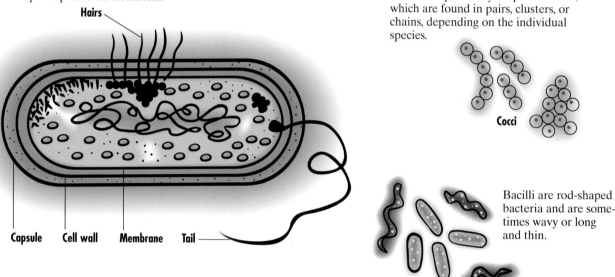

Hairs

Capsule   **Cell wall**   **Membrane**   **Tail**

Cocci are spherically shaped bacteria, which are found in pairs, clusters, or chains, depending on the individual species.

Cocci

Bacilli are rod-shaped bacteria and are sometimes wavy or long and thin.

Bacilli

Fungi

Fungi are more highly advanced than bacteria but not quite as advanced as plants. They come in many varieties of yeasts and molds.

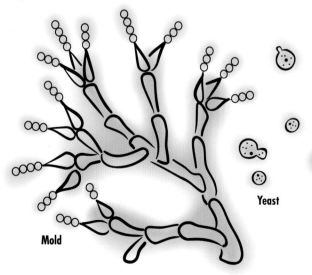

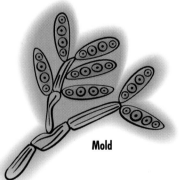

Mold

Yeast

Mold

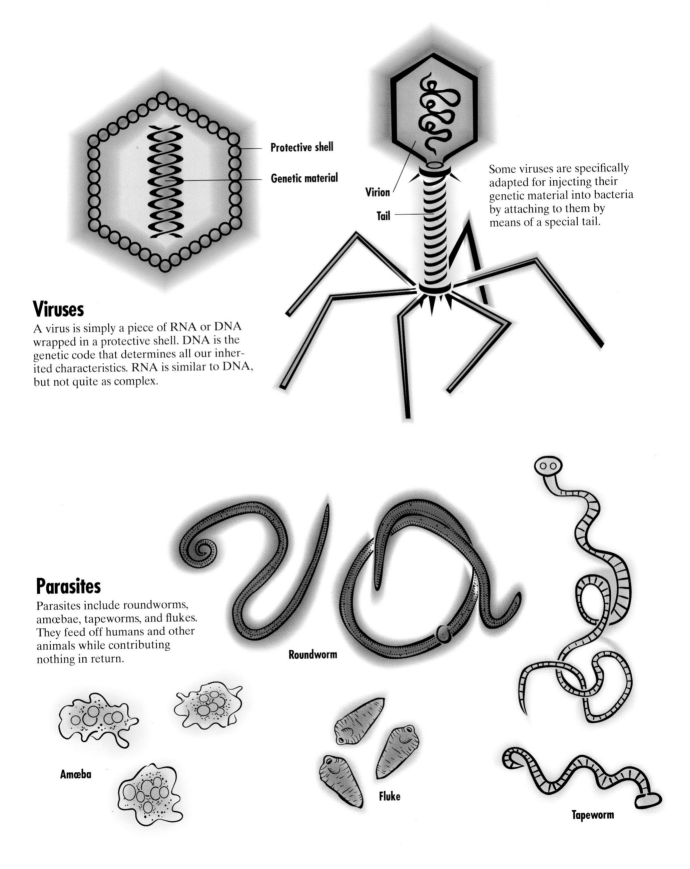

Protective shell

Genetic material

Virion

Tail

Some viruses are specifically adapted for injecting their genetic material into bacteria by attaching to them by means of a special tail.

Viruses

A virus is simply a piece of RNA or DNA wrapped in a protective shell. DNA is the genetic code that determines all our inherited characteristics. RNA is similar to DNA, but not quite as complex.

Parasites

Parasites include roundworms, amœbae, tapeworms, and flukes. They feed off humans and other animals while contributing nothing in return.

Roundworm

Amœba

Fluke

Tapeworm

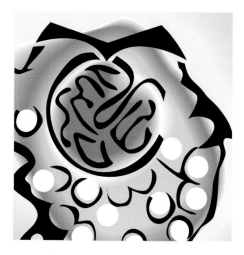

What Are the White Blood Cells?

WE'VE SEEN THAT the white blood cells, which are the backbone of the immune system, come in all shapes and sizes and have many different functions, but they all have three characteristics in common. First, each has a *nucleus*, which is the inner essential part of a cell that contains the material for growth, nourishment, and reproduction. In contrast, red blood cells do not have a nucleus. Second, each serves primarily an immune function, whereas red blood cells exist for the transport of oxygen. Third, all white blood cells arise from the same "parent," called the *stem cell*, which is located in the bone marrow. Stem cells give "birth" to about five different kinds of immature blood cells, which then develop over time until they reach "adulthood." This development phase takes place in different parts of the body, depending on the type of blood cell.

One type of white blood cell that plays a very important role in the immune system is the *T-cell*. The T stands for *thymus*, which is a gland that lies just beneath the sternum (breastbone). When humans are still in the fetal stage of development, the immature T-cells in the bone marrow migrate to the thymus, where they complete the maturation process. While abnormal T-cells are eliminated, each normal T-cell "learns" to respond to a single foreign intruder and is then assigned to a command post in the spleen or lymph nodes; here it remains on alert for an attack by an enemy. (T-cells will be discussed in greater detail in Chapters 8, 10, and 13.)

Another white blood cell essential to immune function is the *B-cell*. Unlike the T-cell, it is not named for a human body part but rather for the organ where immune cell maturation in birds takes place, the *bursa*. No one is sure where B-cell development in humans takes place, but many think it is in the bone marrow. This is convenient for our purposes, for we can think of the B as standing for *b*one marrow. Like T-cells, mature B-cells move to the spleen and lymph nodes to await a call to action. (More on B-cells appears in Chapters 6, 7, and 10.)

When B-cells are activated by foreign invasion, some of them transform into *plasma cells*. These are the B-cells that produce *antibodies*, which are specialized "chemicals" that bind to infectious organisms and signal the immune system to terminate them. B-cells that do not become plasma cells instead remain poised for a rapid response to any future invasion by the same organism.

Another white blood cell that develops in the bone marrow is the *monocyte*. This cell matures very rapidly, then moves into the bloodstream and is carried to the far reaches of the body. Though monocytes appear in large numbers when an infection occurs, their main purpose is to transform into yet another type of white blood cell, the *macrophage*. Macrophages are jumbo-sized cells with ravenous appetites that kill and eat bacteria or old blood cells that have been marked for execution by B-cells, T-cells, or complement (see Chapter 2). Some are free to roam and scavenge, while others remain fixed in the spleen, lymph nodes, bone marrow, lungs, and liver, where they can catch and eat the organisms and cells that float by.

Macrophages are not the only white blood cells that kill and eat bacteria; *neutrophils* also perform this function. Neutrophils typically mature in the bone marrow before venturing out into the blood. A bacterial infection is usually met with increased production of neutrophils by the bone marrow. However, sometimes an infection is so severe that production can't keep up, and immature neutrophils called *bands* spill out into the bloodstream. When a doctor uses an elevated white blood cell count to diagnose a bacterial infection, the doctor is usually referring to an increase in the number of neutrophils.

The term *phagocyte* is generally applied to any cell capable of eating another cell. Neutrophils and macrophages clearly fall into this category. It is also generally agreed that *eosinophils* are phagocytes. Not much is known about eosinophils, but most scientists believe they perform at least two important functions. First, they help regulate the severity of allergic reactions, and second, they kill a number of parasites that may infect the body.

Basophils are relatives of the *mast cell* family and contain all the *histamine* supply of the blood. When a person is exposed to a substance that causes an allergic reaction, such as pollen or dust, mast cells and basophils release histamine. Histamine causes the typical symptoms most people associate with allergies or hayfever. The allergy-causing substance, such as pollen, is called an *allergen*.

In the next chapter, we will examine white blood cell function in more detail and consolidate the different types of white blood cells described above into tidy categories.

The Blood Cell Family Tree

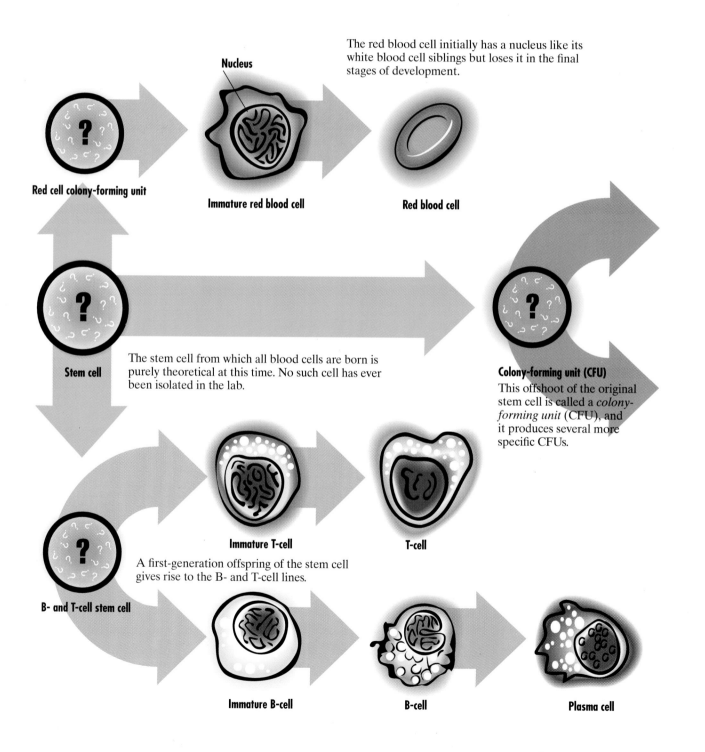

The red blood cell initially has a nucleus like its white blood cell siblings but loses it in the final stages of development.

Nucleus

Red cell colony-forming unit

Immature red blood cell

Red blood cell

Stem cell

The stem cell from which all blood cells are born is purely theoretical at this time. No such cell has ever been isolated in the lab.

Colony-forming unit (CFU)
This offshoot of the original stem cell is called a *colony-forming unit* (CFU), and it produces several more specific CFUs.

Immature T-cell

T-cell

B- and T-cell stem cell

A first-generation offspring of the stem cell gives rise to the B- and T-cell lines.

Immature B-cell

B-cell

Plasma cell

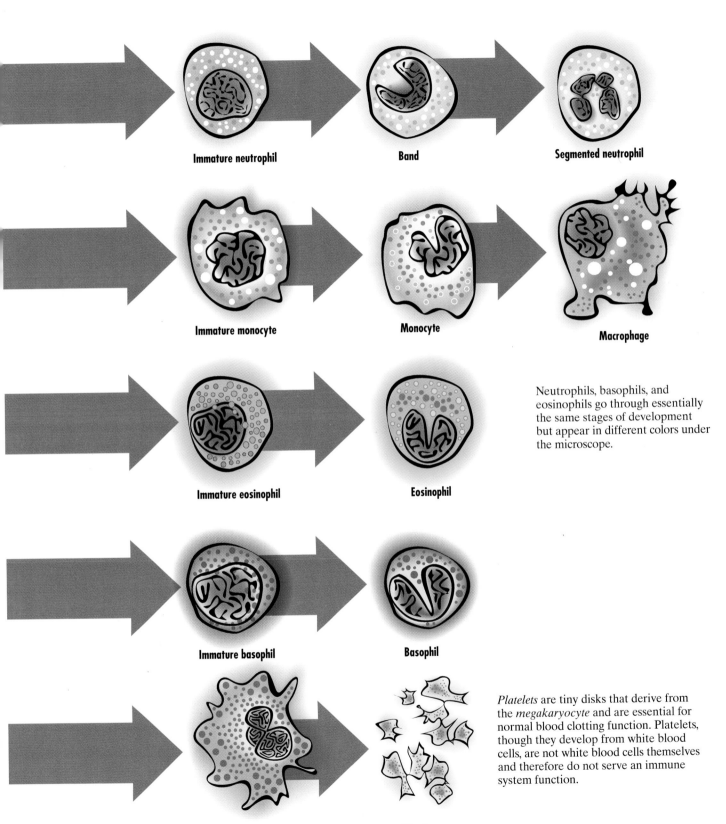

Immature neutrophil

Band

Segmented neutrophil

Immature monocyte

Monocyte

Macrophage

Immature eosinophil

Eosinophil

Neutrophils, basophils, and eosinophils go through essentially the same stages of development but appear in different colors under the microscope.

Immature basophil

Basophil

Megakaryocyte

Platelets

Platelets are tiny disks that derive from the *megakaryocyte* and are essential for normal blood clotting function. Platelets, though they develop from white blood cells, are not white blood cells themselves and therefore do not serve an immune system function.

NOTE For the sake of simplicity, some development steps have been omitted.

B- and T-cell Development

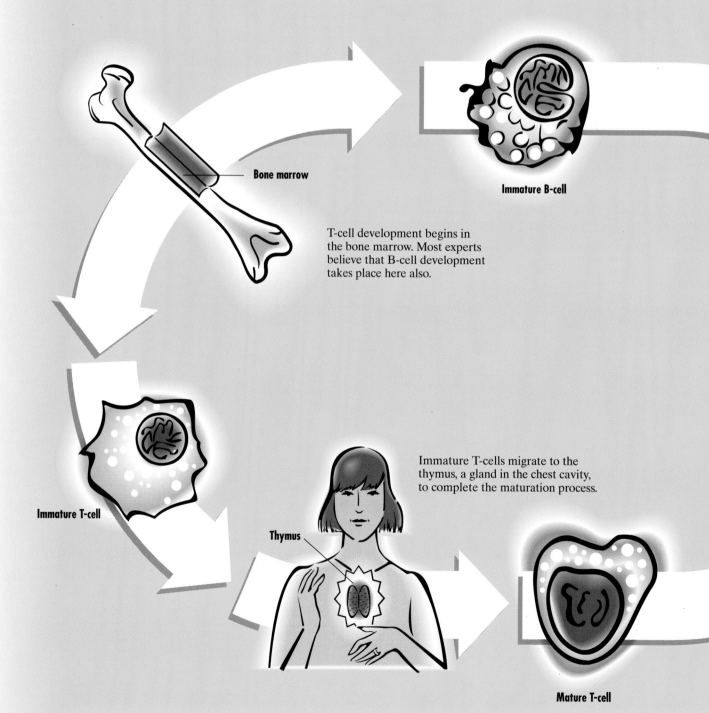

Bone marrow

Immature B-cell

T-cell development begins in the bone marrow. Most experts believe that B-cell development takes place here also.

Immature T-cell

Thymus

Immature T-cells migrate to the thymus, a gland in the chest cavity, to complete the maturation process.

Mature T-cell

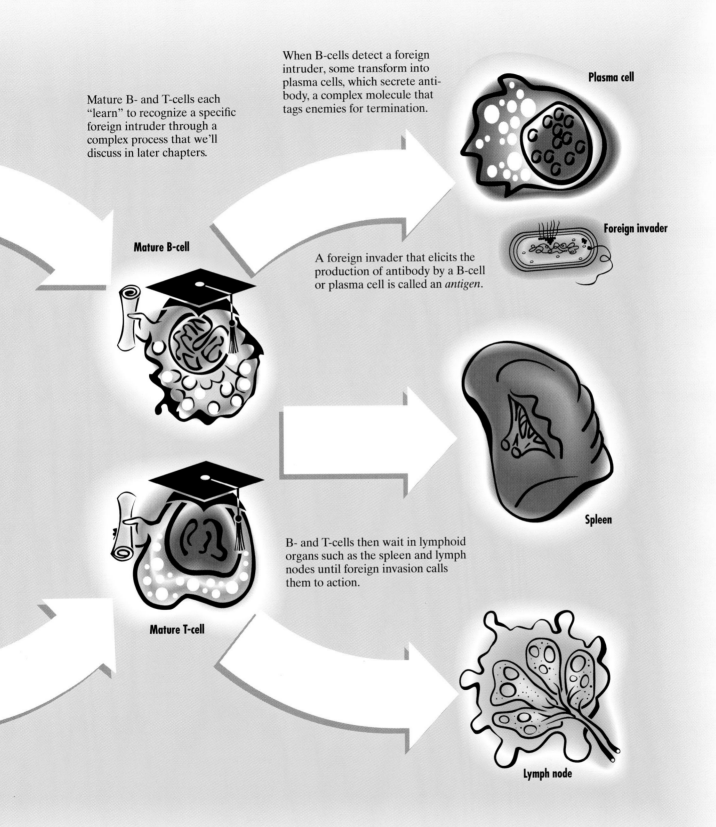

Mature B- and T-cells each "learn" to recognize a specific foreign intruder through a complex process that we'll discuss in later chapters.

When B-cells detect a foreign intruder, some transform into plasma cells, which secrete antibody, a complex molecule that tags enemies for termination.

Plasma cell

Mature B-cell

A foreign invader that elicits the production of antibody by a B-cell or plasma cell is called an *antigen*.

Foreign invader

Spleen

B- and T-cells then wait in lymphoid organs such as the spleen and lymph nodes until foreign invasion calls them to action.

Mature T-cell

Lymph node

The Phagocytes and Granulocytes

Phagocytes

The monocyte's main purpose is to develop into the macrophage, a large phagocyte that eats invading organisms. Some macrophages are free to roam and scavenge, while others are fixed in a position to kill passersby.

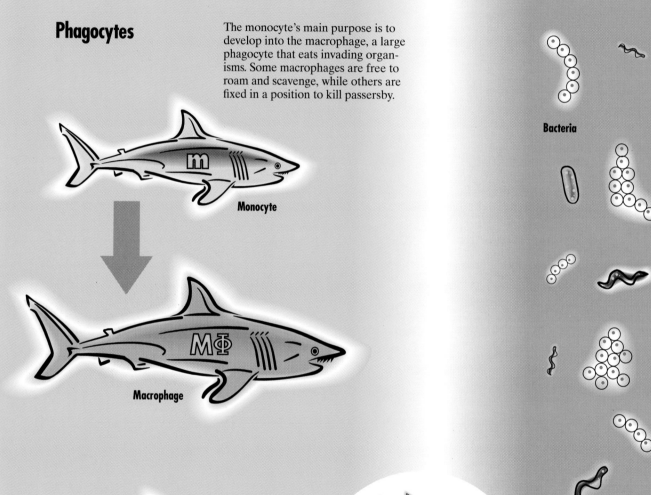

Monocyte

Macrophage

Neutrophil

Bacteria

In a bacterial infection, neutrophils multiply to meet the challenge. Sometimes more of these phagocytes are needed than the bone marrow can supply, and immature neutrophils called bands escape into the blood.

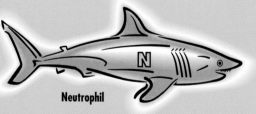

Granulocytes

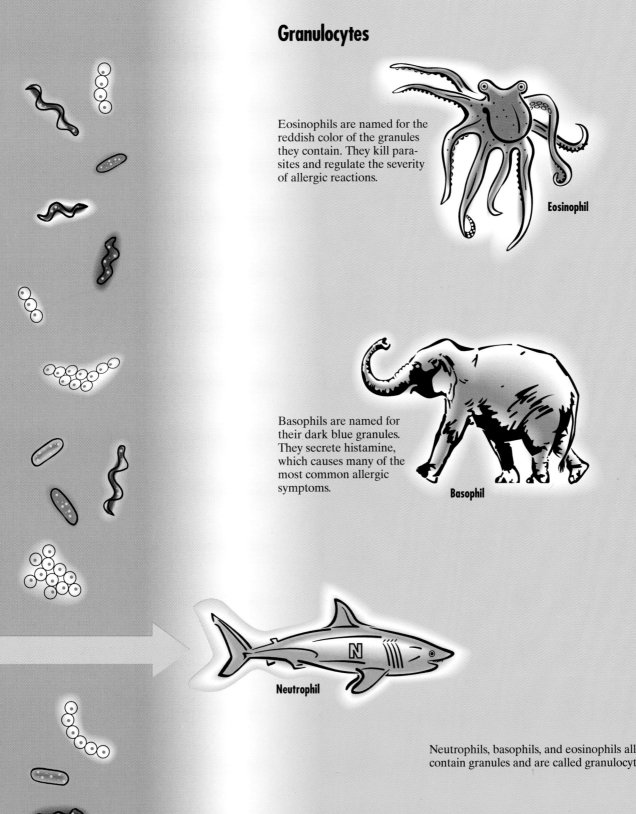

Eosinophils are named for the reddish color of the granules they contain. They kill parasites and regulate the severity of allergic reactions.

Eosinophil

Basophils are named for their dark blue granules. They secrete histamine, which causes many of the most common allergic symptoms.

Basophil

Neutrophil

Neutrophils, basophils, and eosinophils all contain granules and are called granulocytes.

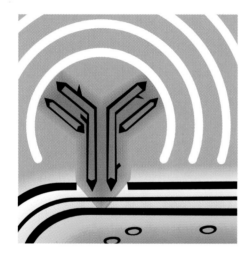

CHAPTER

5

What White Blood Cells Do and How They're Grouped

SO FAR, WE'VE met nine different types of white blood cell. The stem cell is the parent of all blood cells. The T-cell and B-cell play very important roles in immune function that will be covered in Chapters 7 and 8. The plasma cell derives from the B-cell and produces antibodies. The monocyte develops into the macrophage, which, along with the neutrophil, eats bacteria and dead cells. The basophil and the eosinophil both play roles in allergic reactions, and eosinophils also are involved in parasitic infections.

Thus, we have a sense that white blood cells basically perform three functions: they eat foreign invaders, they secrete chemicals that are vital for immune function, and they control how other white cells do their jobs. Not all white blood cells perform all these functions, however. Basophils, for example, secrete histamine, but don't eat or control other cells. Macrophages eat, but don't secrete or control. Eosinophils secrete substances that modify allergic reactions and eat infectious organisms, but don't control other white blood cells. Similarly, T-cells secrete "communication" chemicals and control other cells, but don't eat them.

As we saw in Chapter 2, the white blood cells fall into three broad categories with respect to how they defend the body. The first branch, called *humoral immunity*, is based upon the B-cell and the destruction of foreign invaders by means of antibody secretion. The B-cell population manufactures literally millions of different types of antibody, and each antibody is effective against only one specific enemy. Each B-cell produces a single variety of antibody, which it then displays on its surface as an "antenna," or *receptor*, to detect a particular foreign intruder. When such an organism is identified, the B-cell divides into many identical siblings, or *clones*. Together, they secrete lots of antibody in order to thoroughly coat their target. This then alerts the phagocytes to surround and devour the invader.

The second category of white blood cell is the *cell-mediated immunity* branch. It is based upon the T-cell, which acts as the reconnaissance unit in communicating with and controlling the actions of other immune cells. Like B-cells, T-cells are specific for one particular type of foreign intruder and also wear receptors on their surfaces; however, their antennas are made of protein rather than antibody.

There are several different types of T-cells, and each performs a distinctive function. *Helper T-cells* signal the B-cells to begin secreting antibody in response to a foreign invasion. *Suppressor T-cells* do the opposite: they counteract the stimulatory effects of the helper T-cell. *Killer T-cells*, also called *cytotoxic T-cells,* zero in on cells that have become infected with viruses and kill the whole cells. *Inflammatory T-cells* specialize in attracting inflammatory cells to the site of an infection or injury. As we shall see in Chapter 17, it is the loss of helper and inflammatory T-cells that makes patients with AIDS susceptible to certain infections.

Nonspecific effector cells are the third branch of white blood cells. These cells, unlike B- and T-cells, do not have specific receptors for specific invaders; they are capable of killing many different enemies without outside assistance. The nonspecific effectors include neutrophils and macrophages, which we have met already, and the *natural killer*, or *NK, cells*, which are capable of killing virus-infected cells and bursting cancer cells.

We've now spent five chapters familiarizing ourselves with the players in the immune system and their designated roles. In the next five chapters, we will get an inside look at the continuous workings of each segment of the body's defense department.

Humoral Immunity

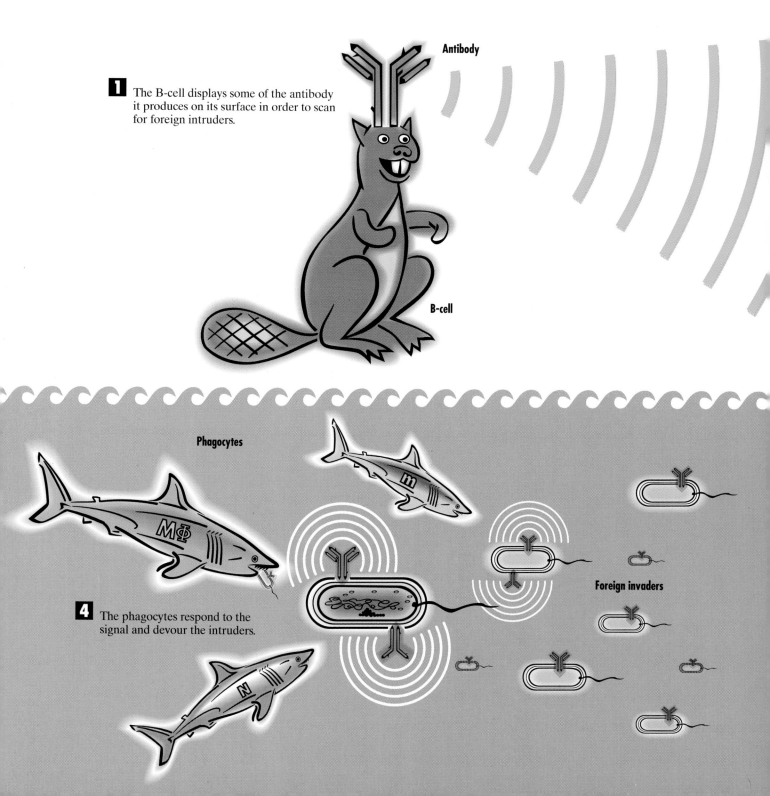

Antibody

1 The B-cell displays some of the antibody it produces on its surface in order to scan for foreign intruders.

B-cell

Phagocytes

4 The phagocytes respond to the signal and devour the intruders.

Foreign invaders

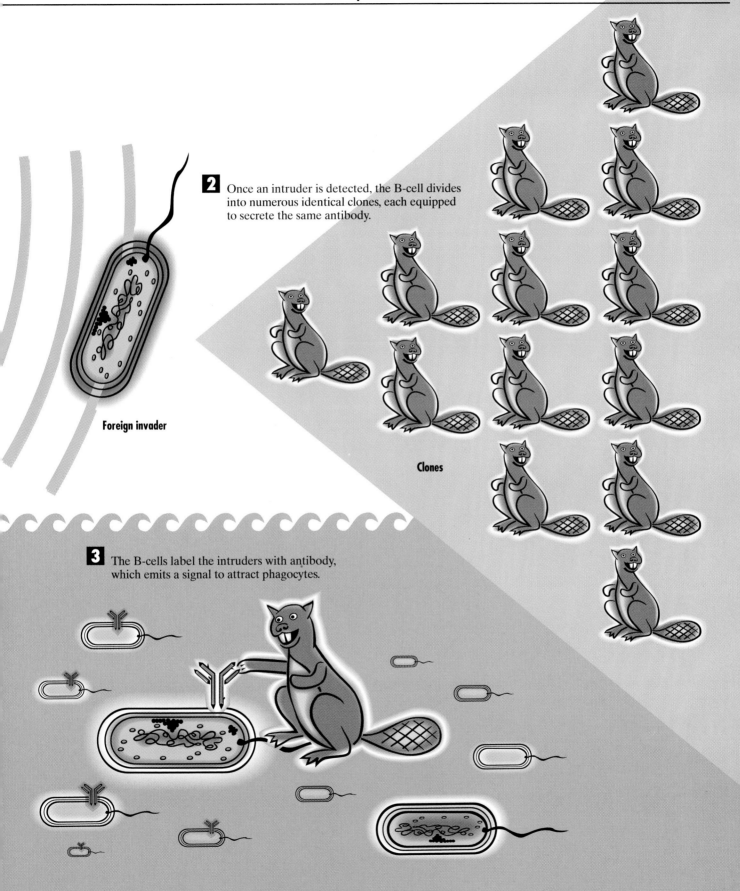

2 Once an intruder is detected, the B-cell divides into numerous identical clones, each equipped to secrete the same antibody.

Foreign invader

Clones

3 The B-cells label the intruders with antibody, which emits a signal to attract phagocytes.

Cell-Mediated Immunity

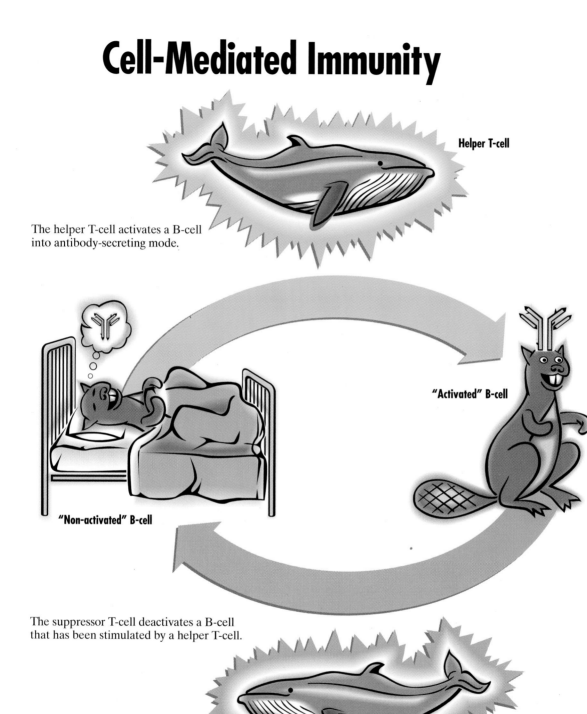

Helper T-cell

The helper T-cell activates a B-cell into antibody-secreting mode.

"Non-activated" B-cell

"Activated" B-cell

The suppressor T-cell deactivates a B-cell that has been stimulated by a helper T-cell.

Suppressor T-cell

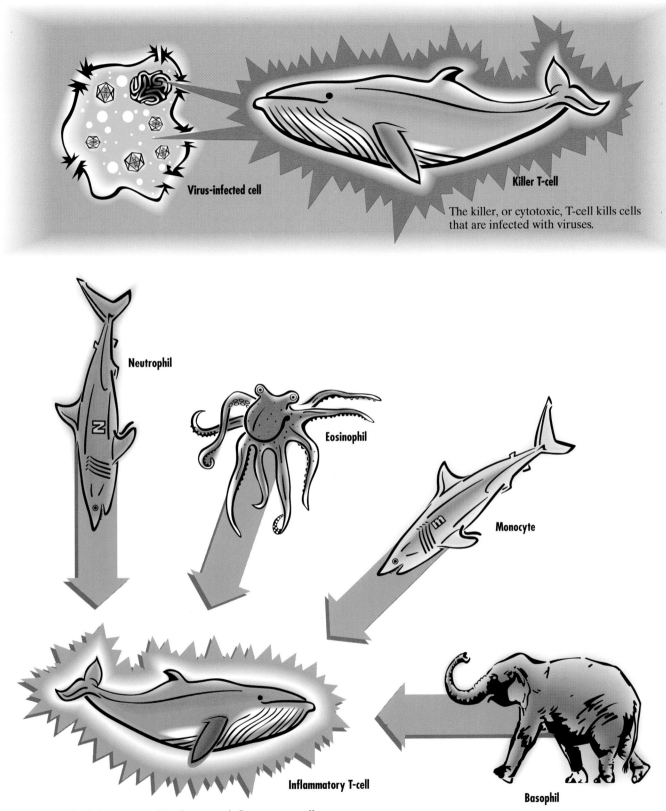

Virus-infected cell

Killer T-cell

The killer, or cytotoxic, T-cell kills cells that are infected with viruses.

Neutrophil

Eosinophil

Monocyte

Inflammatory T-cell

Basophil

The inflammatory T-cell attracts inflammatory cells, such as neutrophils, eosinophils, monocytes, and basophils, to the site of an infection or injury.

Nonspecific Effector Cells

Common targets of the nonspecific effector cells include cancer cells, bacteria, and body cells that have been infiltrated by viruses.

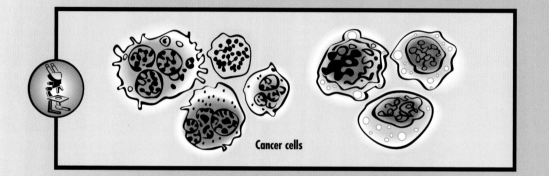

Cancer cells

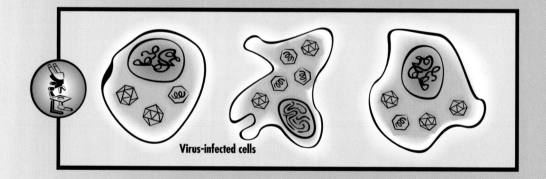

Virus-infected cells

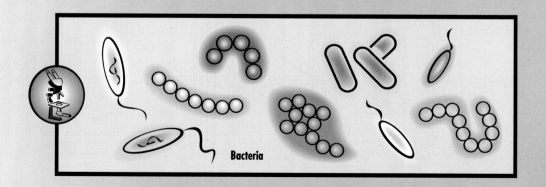

Bacteria

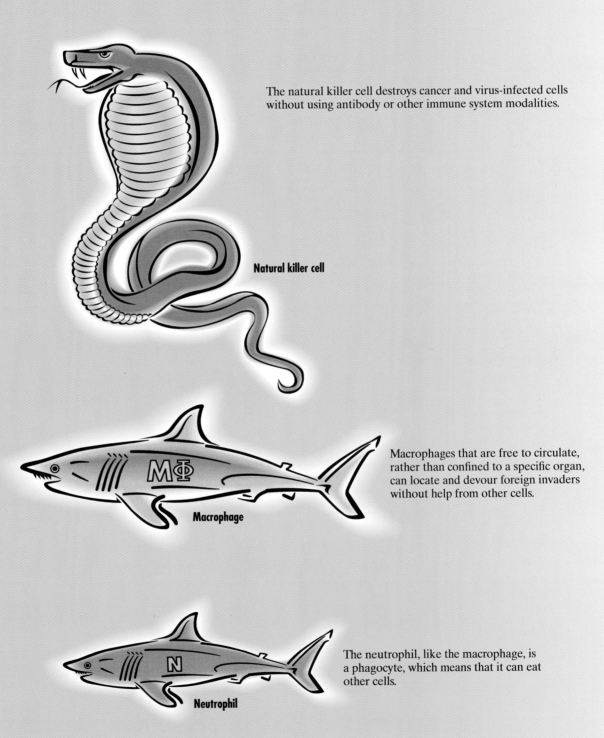

The natural killer cell destroys cancer and virus-infected cells without using antibody or other immune system modalities.

Natural killer cell

Macrophages that are free to circulate, rather than confined to a specific organ, can locate and devour foreign invaders without help from other cells.

Macrophage

The neutrophil, like the macrophage, is a phagocyte, which means that it can eat other cells.

Neutrophil

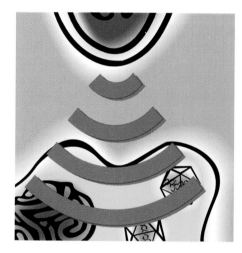

How the Immune System Identifies Intruders

I N THE PREVIOUS chapter, we learned that detection of a foreign invader is a crucial step in the body's defense of itself. But how exactly do the cells of the immune system know what doesn't belong? Since foreign intruders come in so many varieties, is there also a variety of ways in which to recognize them? Are we born with these recognition abilities, or do they develop only after an encounter with the enemy?

To begin, the immune system is able to identify certain organisms as being foreign because they look different from other cells. Bacteria, for example, are made of certain proteins that simply are not seen in normal body tissues, while viruses are recognized because the genetic code they carry is unique. The "antennas," or receptors, present on the surfaces of B- and T-cells are specifically designed to detect these characteristics. B-cells and the antibodies they secrete are especially adept at catching intruders like bacteria, which usually are found outside of other cells. T-cells specialize in identifying viruses and other organisms that invade the inner workings of body cells.

B-cells and T-cells depend on an initial exposure to the enemy before they can mount an attack. As we'll see in later chapters, these cells must be presented with a specific antigen, usually by a macrophage, before they can multiply, defeat the enemy, and linger in the form of *memory cells* to provide long-term protection. This is a time-consuming process; therefore, some form of defense is necessary during the initial stages of a foreign invasion. The *complement system* accomplishes this function.

Complement is a substance found in the blood that can bind to the surface of any cell, be it a bacterium or a normal body cell, and attract phagocytes such as neutrophils and macrophages to destroy it. Complement can also kill cells on its own by punching holes in the cells' outer membranes, which allows enough water in to cause the cells to actually burst. Normal body cells, however, are protected with special equipment that deactivates complement's effects, so only cells that aren't welcome are vulnerable to attacks by the complement system.

Still, some bacteria are crafty and have developed ways to penetrate the complement barricade. Fortunately, all the body's defenses have backup systems, and complement is no exception. When such resistant bacteria do manage to slip by, they are spotted by macrophages that are continuously on the prowl. The macrophages send a message to the liver, which quickly manufactures a substance that can bind to the bacteria and change their shape. Complement can then treat this deformed invader as an entirely new organism and call in the phagocytes to do their job.

While the complement system is our inborn means of recognizing the enemy, we also depend on other components that can adjust to the body's changing needs. In Chapter 5, we learned that the B-cell uses antibodies mounted on its surface in order to detect intruders. We also learned that each B-cell produces only one type of antibody, which, in turn, is effective against only one type of foreign invader. How, then, are B-cells able to recognize millions upon millions of different enemies?

The key lies in our genetic makeup. The *DNA* that makes us who we are, that defines our eye and hair color, our size and shape, and everything else that is inherited, also determines our antibody-making ability. We inherit this ability in the form of "puzzle pieces" that can be reassembled in different ways, depending on the needs of different B-cells. In addition, the "glues" that are used to put the pieces together can vary extensively. This alone allows for a staggering degree of variation, but it doesn't end here. The antibody-making machinery within the B-cell can *mutate*, or change, into an entirely new factory, capable of producing a completely different antibody type. All this adds up to a tremendous potential for diversity.

The innate complement system and the adaptive antibody system work hand-in-hand. The binding of complement to a bacterium can increase the production of antibody by the B-cell. Conversely, the binding of antibody to an organism can activate the complement system. It is a perfect example of different segments of the immune system combining their efforts for the common good.

Recognition of and Specificity for Different Enemies

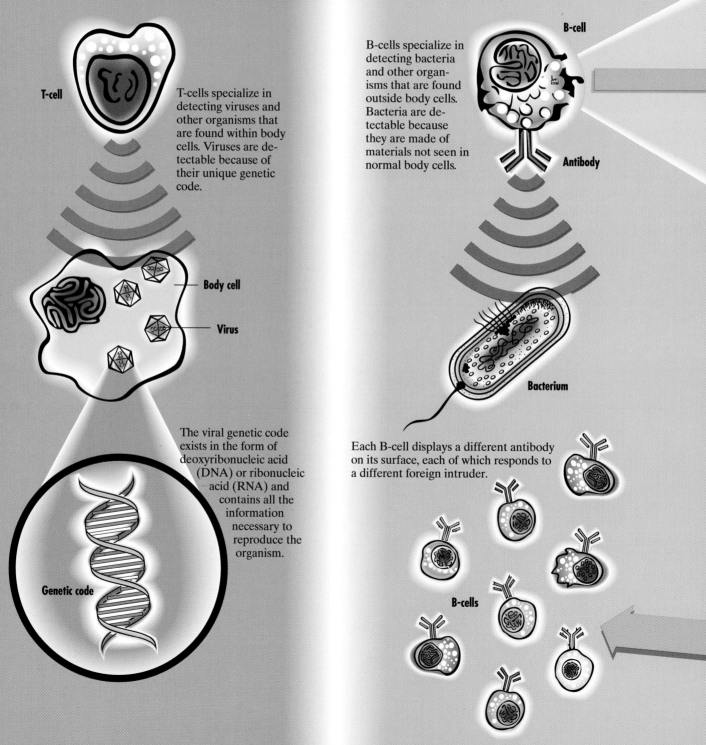

T-cell

T-cells specialize in detecting viruses and other organisms that are found within body cells. Viruses are detectable because of their unique genetic code.

B-cell

B-cells specialize in detecting bacteria and other organisms that are found outside body cells. Bacteria are detectable because they are made of materials not seen in normal body cells.

Antibody

Body cell

Virus

Bacterium

The viral genetic code exists in the form of deoxyribonucleic acid (DNA) or ribonucleic acid (RNA) and contains all the information necessary to reproduce the organism.

Each B-cell displays a different antibody on its surface, each of which responds to a different foreign intruder.

Genetic code

B-cells

The antibody-making "factories" are distributed amongst the B-cells in the form of "puzzle pieces."

The "puzzle pieces" are reassembled within each B-cell using a variety of different "glues."

The antibody-making "factory" within each B-cell can also mutate into an entirely different "factory," capable of producing a whole new antibody.

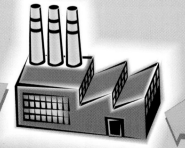
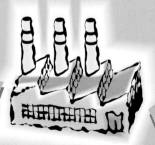

Complement in Action

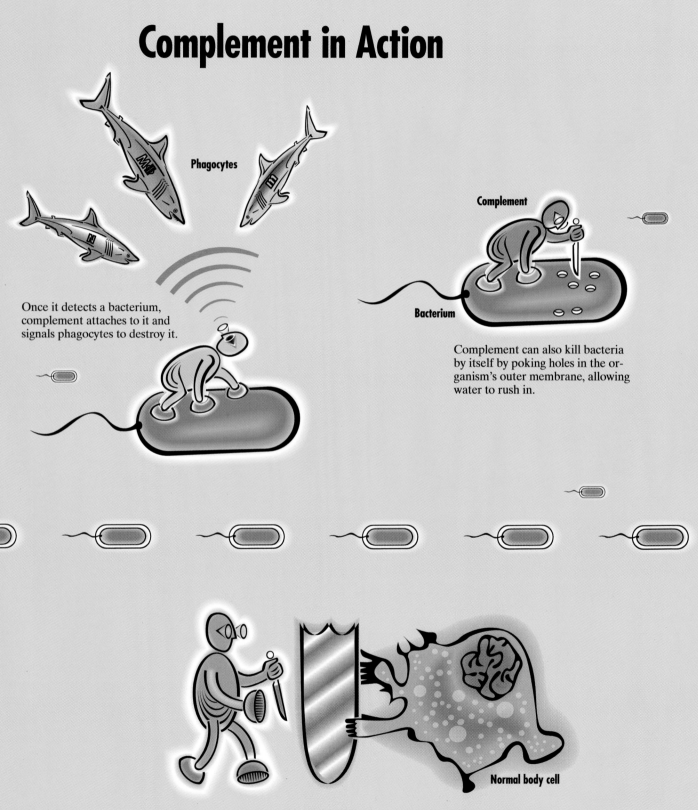

Phagocytes

Once it detects a bacterium, complement attaches to it and signals phagocytes to destroy it.

Complement

Bacterium

Complement can also kill bacteria by itself by poking holes in the organism's outer membrane, allowing water to rush in.

Normal body cell

Normal body cells have special proteins on their outer membranes that protect them from an attack by complement.

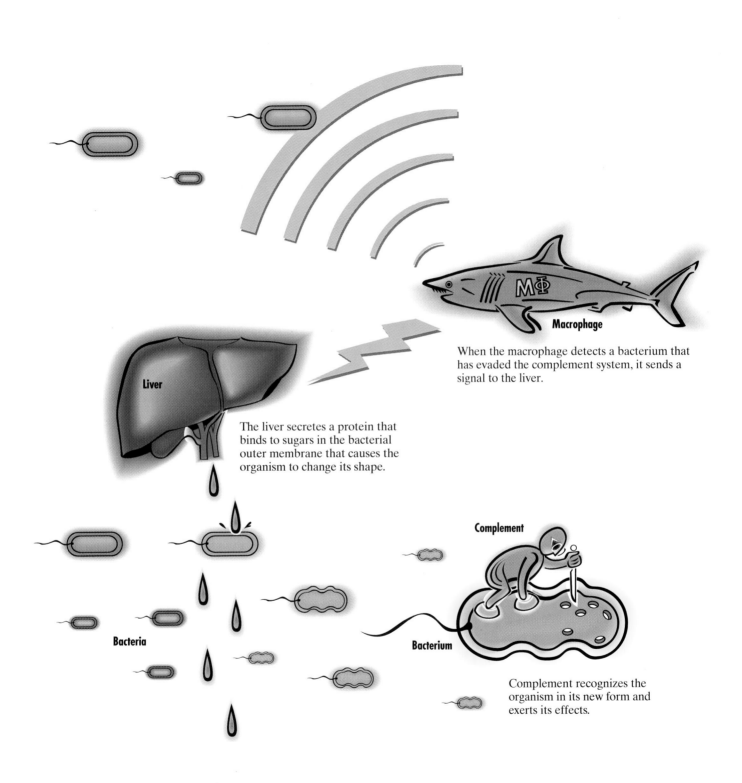

Macrophage

When the macrophage detects a bacterium that has evaded the complement system, it sends a signal to the liver.

Liver

The liver secretes a protein that binds to sugars in the bacterial outer membrane that causes the organism to change its shape.

Complement

Bacteria

Bacterium

Complement recognizes the organism in its new form and exerts its effects.

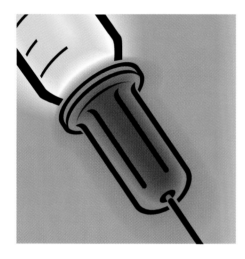

7

The B-Cell, Antibodies, and Vaccines

NOW THAT WE know a bit about the B-cell and what it does, we can explore some of the more intricate details of the humoral immunity system. In this chapter, we will learn about B-cell development and how the body ensures that only normal cells are released into circulation. We will also examine the different types of antibodies secreted by B-cells and plasma cells and see how this technology is used in the treatment and prevention of various diseases.

Like all other blood cells, the B-cell derives from the *stem cell*. Once the stem cell has produced an immature descendant, it is incumbent upon the *stromal cells* of the bone marrow to decide whether it will mature into a B-cell or another cell type. Any cell that is designated as a new B-cell must then receive a second signal from a specialized structure called the *surrogate complex*, whose responsibility it is to determine which B-cells are permitted to survive and circulate throughout the immune system. The surrogate complex is remarkably adept at not allowing abnormal cells to escape the bone marrow; B-cells that are immature, that have receptors which recognize normal body structures, or that are abnormal for any reason, are promptly sentenced to death. (More on cells that target "self" organs will appear in Chapter 13.) Once a B-cell has received the seal of approval from the stromal cells and surrogate complex, it is released to the spleen and lymph nodes to await its call to action.

The B-cell is activated when detection of a foreign invader is coupled with a signal from *helper T-cells*. When this occurs, a portion of the B-cell contingent transforms rapidly into *plasma cells*, which secrete antibodies, mostly of the *IgM* type, to fight off the intruder. Ig stands for *immunoglobulin*, which is another word for antibody. The remaining B-cells become *memory B-cells*, which, as their name suggests, remember the particular foreign intruder and remain on alert for future invasions. Should the same enemy launch a subsequent attack, the memory B-cells are able to respond with much greater efficiency by multiplying and producing antibodies, mostly of the *IgG* type, and by transforming into plasma cells.

The antibodies produced by B-cells and plasma cells come in five different varieties. The *IgM* type, as we have seen, is the first to appear when the body is invaded by an enemy. It attaches to the intruder and signals phagocytes to destroy it; its effects are short-lived, however. For long-term protection, the body relies on *IgG* antibody. This is the most abundant antibody type, and it provides lifelong immunity against a particular enemy after an initial attack has been effectively suppressed. It is also the only immunoglobulin that can pass through the placenta of a pregnant mother in order to provide her fetus with immunity. *IgA* antibody is found in nasal, intestinal, vaginal, and prostatic secretions, as well as in tears, saliva, and early breast milk, and gives these fluids much of their ability to fight off intruders before they enter the body. *IgE* antibody, as we shall see in Chapter 11, is seen in allergic reactions and parasitic infections. Scientists have yet to discover the function served by the last antibody type, *IgD*. Putting all these antibody types together spells "DAMaGE" for the enemy, giving us an easy way to remember them!

Allowing the immune system to meet an intruder and form a response works well if the illness caused by that intruder is a minor one; this process is called *active immunization*. But what if that illness is a serious one, such as polio? Even after the initial infection has been defeated and long-term immunity has been established, the possibility of lifelong paralysis remains. Wouldn't it be better if immunity could be given before a person suffered the actual disease?

This is where *vaccines* enter the picture. A vaccine is a form of active immunization in which an infectious organism injected into the body causes the immune system to make antibodies and activate T-cells against the organism without causing the full-blown disease. There are basically two types of viral vaccines: those containing "killed" virus and those containing live, but weakened, virus. The latter has the advantage of requiring not only a shorter time period but also a smaller amount of the organism in order to provide immunity. The disadvantage is that it can cause a mild form of the illness it is designed to prevent, whereas the "killed" vaccine does not. In addition to viral infections, prevention of a select number of bacterial infections can be obtained through vaccination.

Vaccines are available against a wide variety of illnesses. Examples of "killed" virus vaccines include flu, hepatitis B, and rabies. Polio and measles/mumps/rubella (MMR) are examples of vaccines made from live, weakened virus. The diphtheria/pertussis/tetanus (DPT) vaccine is made from the toxins produced by these three bacteria. The pneumococcal pneumonia, *Hemophilus influenzæ* B (HiB), and bacterial meningitis vaccines are all made from sugars taken from the capsules of these bacteria. The protection provided by vaccines can diminish over time, but future exposures to the particular enemy are met with swift retaliation and renewed immunity.

Vaccines

Live, weakened viral vaccines
Measles/mumps/rubella (MMR)
Polio
Smallpox
Killed viral vaccines
Influenza
Hepatitis B
Rabies
Bacterial vaccines
Diphtheria/pertussis/tetanus (DPT)
Pneumococcus (pneumonia)
Meningococcus (meningitis)
Hemophilus influenzæ B (HiB)
Cholera
Typhoid fever

Development of Humoral Immunity

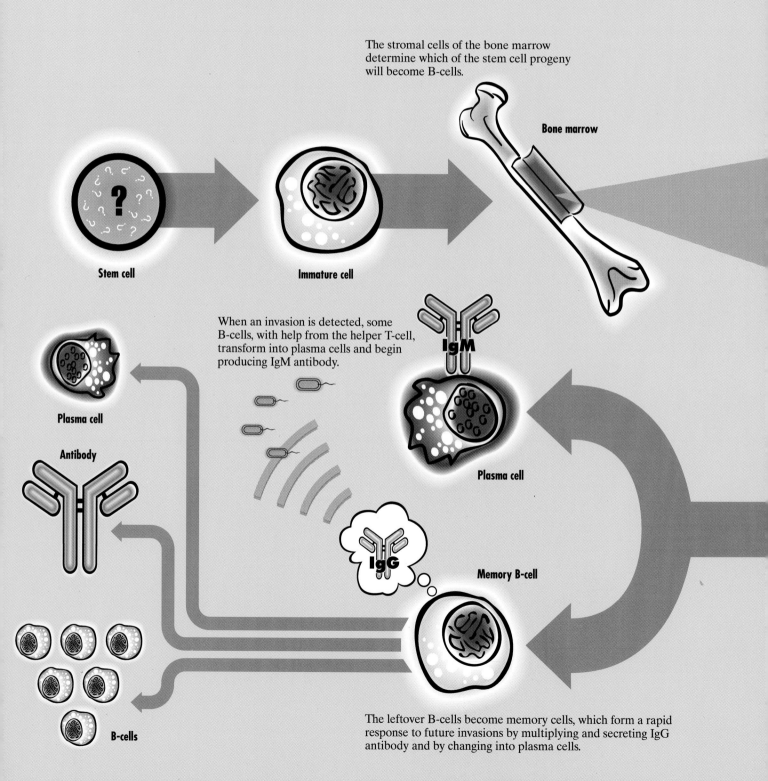

The stromal cells of the bone marrow determine which of the stem cell progeny will become B-cells.

Bone marrow

Stem cell

Immature cell

When an invasion is detected, some B-cells, with help from the helper T-cell, transform into plasma cells and begin producing IgM antibody.

IgM

Plasma cell

Plasma cell

Antibody

IgG

Memory B-cell

B-cells

The leftover B-cells become memory cells, which form a rapid response to future invasions by multiplying and secreting IgG antibody and by changing into plasma cells.

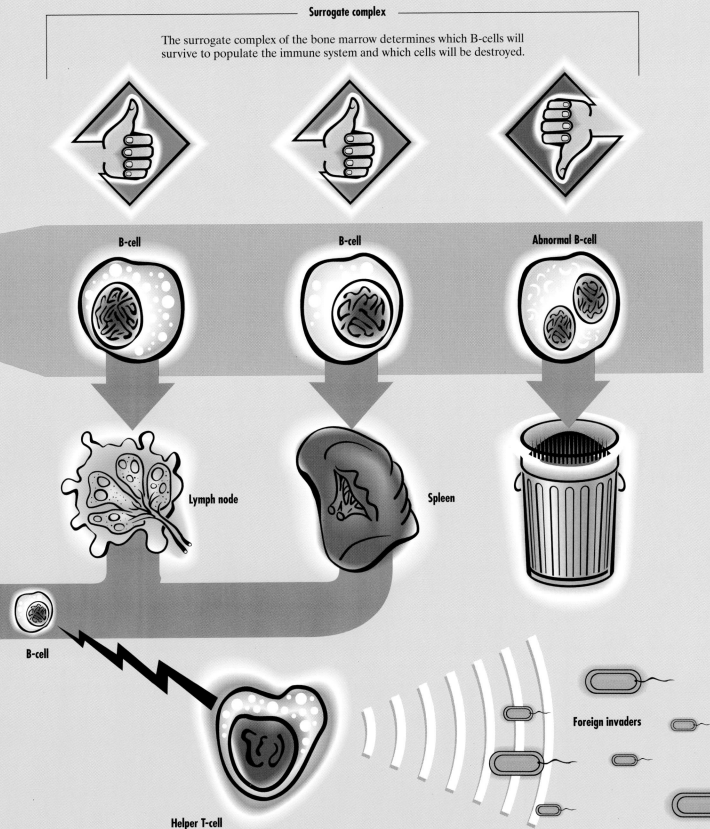

Surrogate complex

The surrogate complex of the bone marrow determines which B-cells will survive to populate the immune system and which cells will be destroyed.

B-cell

B-cell

Abnormal B-cell

Lymph node

Spleen

B-cell

Helper T-cell

Foreign invaders

Antibody Types

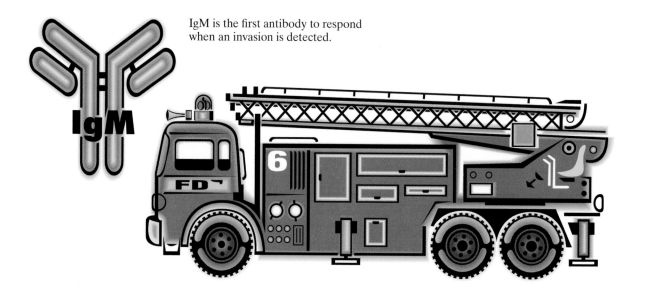

IgM is the first antibody to respond when an invasion is detected.

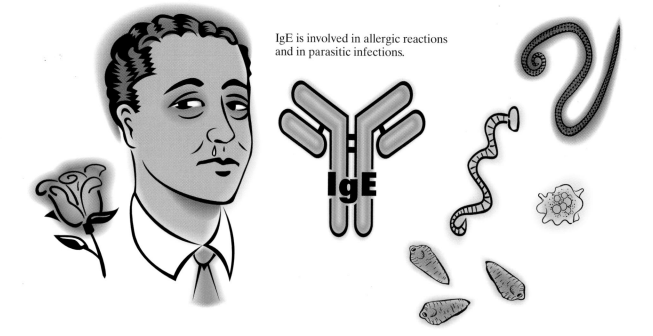

IgE is involved in allergic reactions and in parasitic infections.

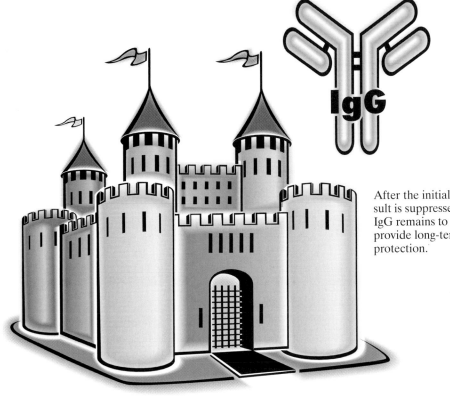

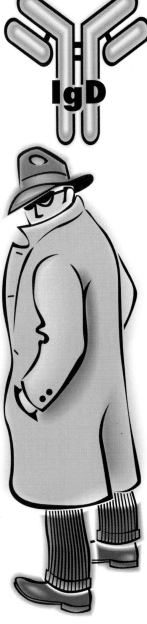

After the initial insult is suppressed, IgG remains to provide long-term protection.

No one knows what IgD does.

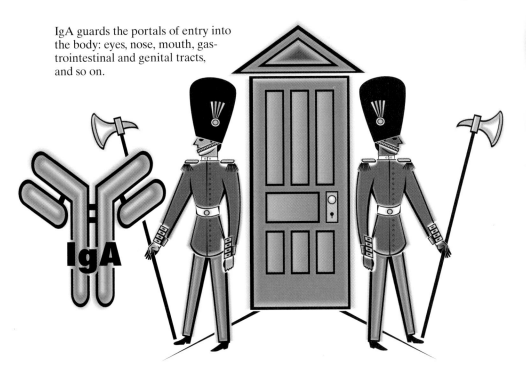

IgA guards the portals of entry into the body: eyes, nose, mouth, gastrointestinal and genital tracts, and so on.

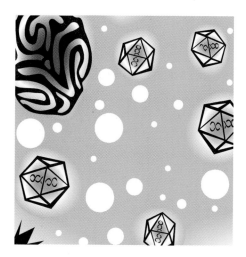

The T-Cell and Cell-Mediated Immunity

T IS ONLY logical to follow a chapter devoted to humoral immunity with one covering cell-mediated immunity. This chapter will expand upon what we already know about the T-cell. We will discuss its development, its various subtypes, and the methods it uses to identify and destroy foreign invaders.

The T-cell, like all blood cells, is borne by the *stem cell*. Immature stem cell products migrate to the *thymus*, a gland located in the chest cavity, where they become T-cell "parents." The progeny generated by these cells must then, like their B-cell counterparts, endure a selection procedure that weeds out T-cells which are abnormal or which have receptors that recognize normal body structures. Each prospective T-cell is tested against a segment of human DNA called the *major histocompatibility complex*, or *MHC*, which makes two varieties of highly complex molecules. Cells binding *class I MHC* molecules, which are found in virtually all body cell types, develop into *killer* (also called *cytotoxic*) or *suppressor T-cells*. Cells that bind to *Class II MHC* molecules, which are found only in immune system cells, move on to become *helper* or *inflammatory T-cells*. Those cells unable to join with either MHC type are given the death penalty. All this occurs while we are still in the fetal stage of development.

Individual T-cells that pass the screening process are, like their B-cell brethren, each programmed to respond to a single enemy. They then join the B-cells in the lymph nodes and spleen, where they wait for a foreign invasion to call them to active duty. When an intruder attacks, it is detected by the *helper T-cell*, which then proceeds to orchestrate a complex, multilayered immune response that includes stimulating B-cells to secrete antibody, signaling *killer T-cells* to destroy infected cells, and alerting *inflammatory T-cells* to call in phagocytes to devour the enemy. Once the incursion has been controlled, the remaining helper T-cells persist as *memory T-cells*, which, like memory B-cells, remain poised to counter any future attacks by the same antigen.

Cell-mediated immunity is active in a variety of circumstances, including transplant rejection, which we will discuss in Chapter 16, and certain types of allergic reactions, which will be covered in Chapter 12. Its most important duty, however, is the containment of infection. As we learned earlier, T-cells specialize in combating organisms like viruses, which penetrate a cell's interior to reach the genetic machinery they need in order to reproduce. But how do T-cells reach viruses that are buried deep within other cells? The answer arrives courtesy of the MHC.

The MHC manufactures transport molecules that deliver organisms to the surfaces of the cells they infect, so that they can be "seen" by immune cells. When a Class I MHC molecule spots a virus using a cell's genetic code for its own procreation, it takes a piece of the virus and moves to the surface of the cell to flag down the appropriate killer T-cell. The T-cell then destroys the entire infected cell by punching holes in its outer membrane or by convincing the cell to commit suicide, a process known as *apoptosis*. Obviously, eradicating whole cells can be costly if the virus spreads from cell to cell faster than the immune system can respond. Such is the case in certain chronic viral infections. In people who carry the hepatitis B virus, for example, progressive cell damage can lead to eventual destruction of the entire liver.

The Class II MHC molecule is also involved in cell-mediated immunity, usually in fighting bacteria. Tuberculosis bacteria, for example, infect the inner workings of macrophages, where they become comfortably isolated within multiple tiny "packages," or *vesicles*. A Class II MHC molecule identifies the organism and brings a piece of it to the cell surface, where an inflammatory T-cell "sees" it and stimulates the macrophage to digest all such organisms contained within its vesicles. This same scenario applies to certain parasites that take up residence within cells of the body.

The cell-mediated immunity unit described above acts in concert with the humoral system depicted in the previous chapter. We have already seen a simplified version of how the helper T-cell assists the B-cell in secreting antibody, but now we can address the MHC's role in this process. When a B-cell's "antenna" detects a foreign intruder, that B-cell binds to it, seals it in a vesicle, and breaks it into pieces. A Class II MHC molecule takes a piece and transports it to the B-cell surface, where a helper T-cell can recognize it and signal the B-cell to secrete antibody.

Cell-Mediated Immunity

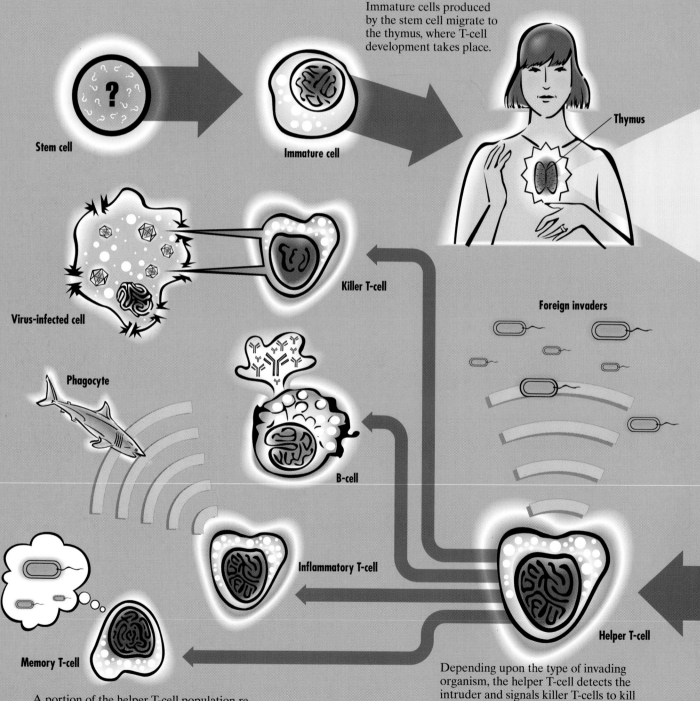

Immature cells produced by the stem cell migrate to the thymus, where T-cell development takes place.

Thymus

Stem cell

Immature cell

Virus-infected cell

Killer T-cell

Foreign invaders

Phagocyte

B-cell

Inflammatory T-cell

Helper T-cell

Memory T-cell

A portion of the helper T-cell population remains in the form of memory cells, for rapid response to suppress future invasions.

Depending upon the type of invading organism, the helper T-cell detects the intruder and signals killer T-cells to kill virus-infected cells, B-cells to secrete antibody, or inflammatory T-cells to summon phagocytes.

Cells that bind with the class I MHC become killer (cytotoxic) or suppressor T-cells. Cells that bind with the class II MHC become helper or inflammatory T-cells. Cells unable to bind with either are destroyed.

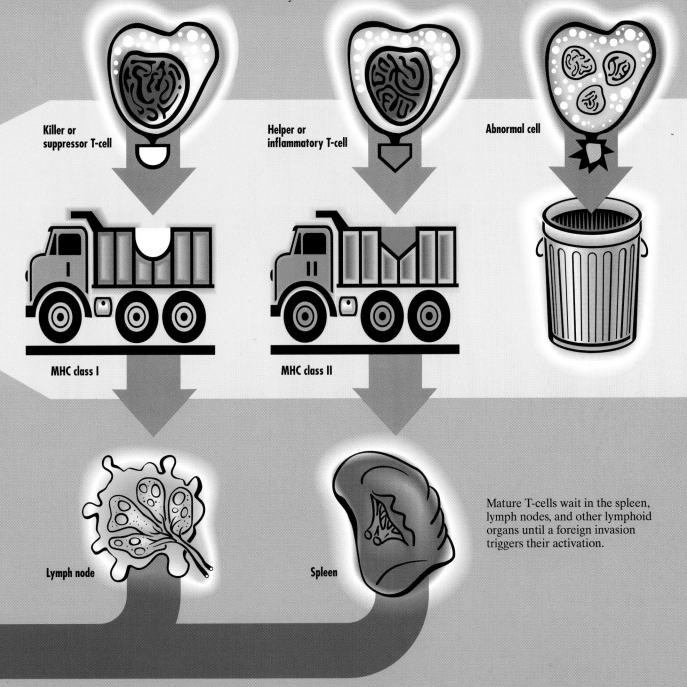

Killer or suppressor T-cell

Helper or inflammatory T-cell

Abnormal cell

MHC class I

MHC class II

Lymph node

Spleen

Mature T-cells wait in the spleen, lymph nodes, and other lymphoid organs until a foreign invasion triggers their activation.

The Major Histocompatibility Complex in Cell-Mediated Immunity

MHC Class I

When the MHC detects a viral infection within a body cell, it carries a piece of the organism to the surface of the cell.

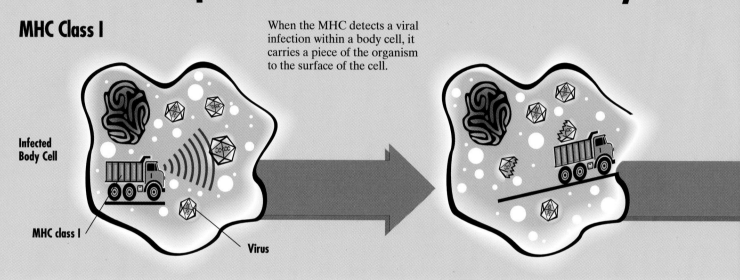

Infected Body Cell

MHC class I

Virus

MHC Class II

When the MHC detects a tuberculosis (TB) infection in vesicles within a macrophage, it carries a piece of the organism to the surface of the cell.

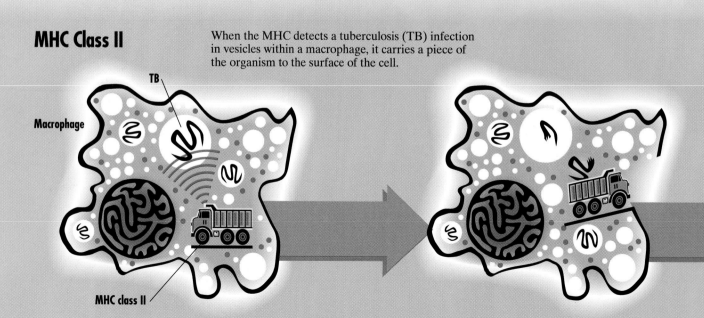

TB

Macrophage

MHC class II

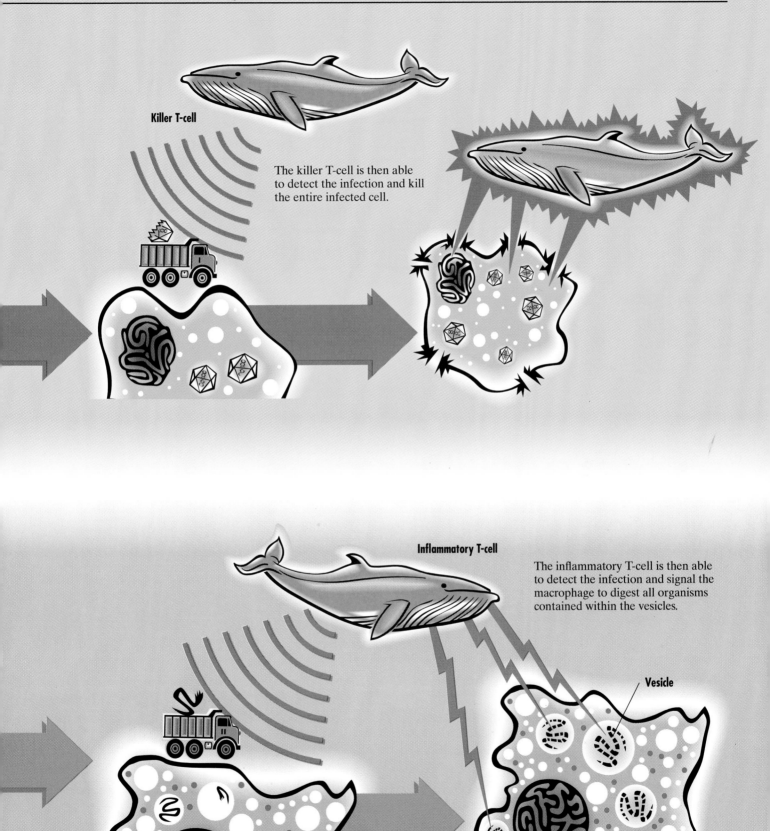

The killer T-cell is then able to detect the infection and kill the entire infected cell.

Killer T-cell

Inflammatory T-cell

The inflammatory T-cell is then able to detect the infection and signal the macrophage to digest all organisms contained within the vesicles.

Vesicle

The Major Histocompatibility Complex in Humoral Immunity

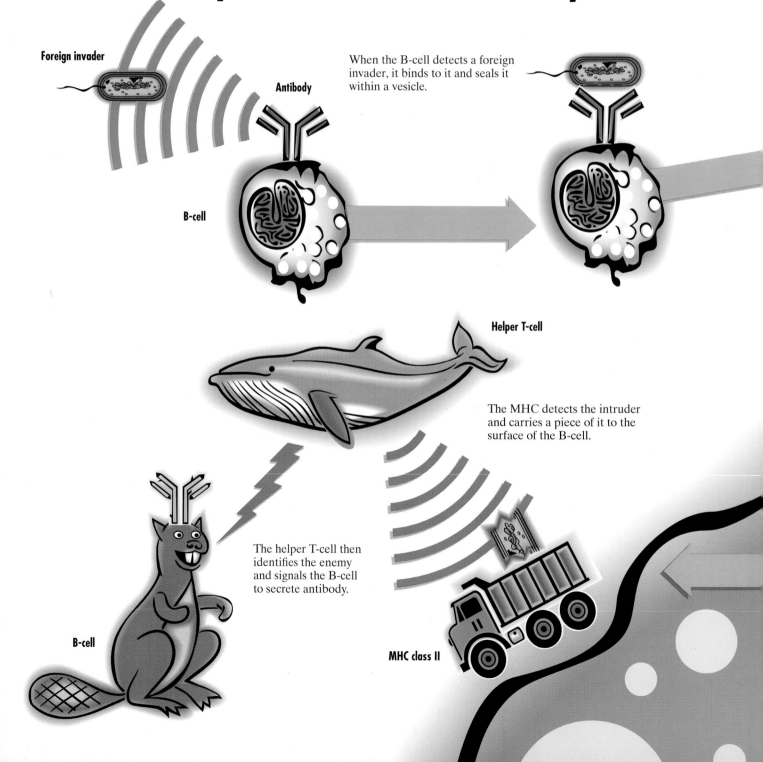

Foreign invader

Antibody

B-cell

When the B-cell detects a foreign invader, it binds to it and seals it within a vesicle.

Helper T-cell

The MHC detects the intruder and carries a piece of it to the surface of the B-cell.

The helper T-cell then identifies the enemy and signals the B-cell to secrete antibody.

B-cell

MHC class II

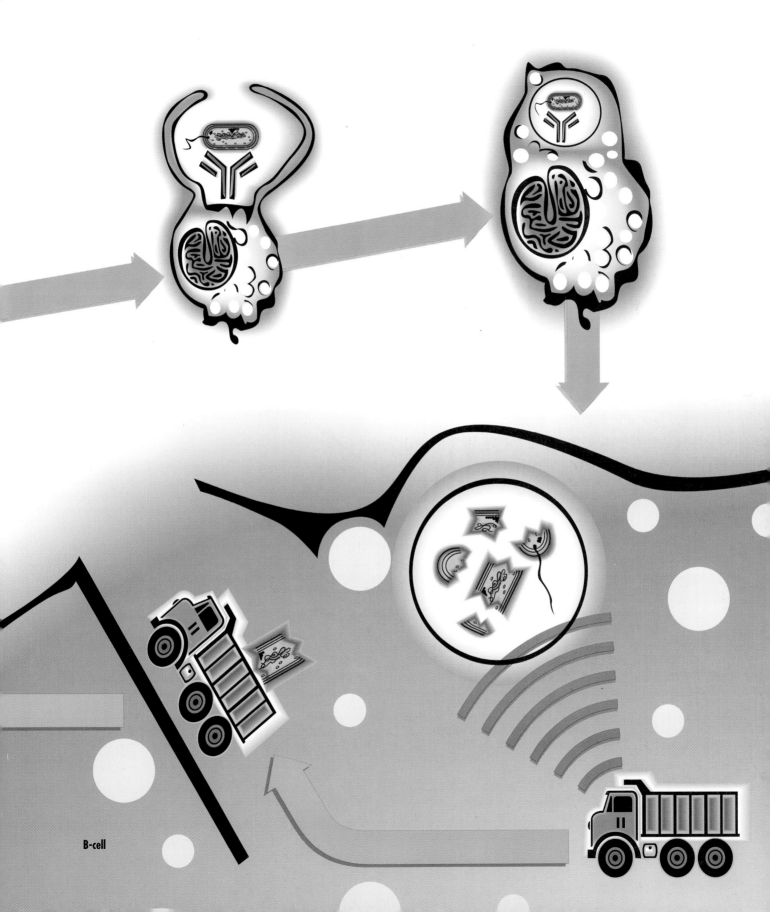

B-cell

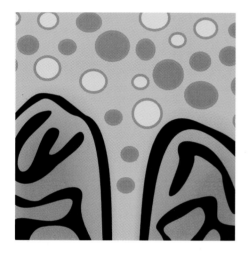

Alternative Classifications of White Blood Cells

AFTER READING ALL these chapters about white blood cells, you might get the impression that the boundaries we've used to categorize them are sharply defined. On the contrary, the delineation is far from distinct, and a great deal of overlapping is involved. Just as a lemon can simultaneously be assigned to a list of fruits, of things that are yellow, or of words beginning with "l," so can white blood cells occupy more than one category at the same time. Let's look at some of these alternative classifications.

We have already touched upon one such grouping, the *phagocytes*. These cells, which are capable of devouring other cells, include the neutrophil, monocyte, macrophage, and probably eosinophil. When an invading organism has been tagged for termination by antibody or complement, it adheres to the surface of a phagocyte summoned to the scene. The enemy is drawn inward as the phagocyte's membrane wraps around it, until it is completely sealed within a bubble called a *phagocytic vacuole*. This engulfing process is called *invagination*. The vacuole then collides with a package of powerful digestive chemicals called a *lysosome*, and the two fuse together. The digestive chemicals are released onto the foreign invader, which is quickly killed and digested. The whole process of swallowing and digestion by phagocytes is called *phagocytosis*.

The phagocytes is not the only group to which the neutrophil and eosinophil belong. Along with the basophil, they also occupy the *granulocyte* category. These cells, as their name suggests, contain granules that accomplish various tasks. The granules of the basophil and its noncirculating relative, the *mast cell*, contain *histamine*, which causes the symptoms commonly associated with allergic reactions; *heparin*, a "blood thinner" that increases a person's tendency to bleed; and some additional chemicals designed to attract other immune cells to an area of illness or injury. The neutrophil's granules contain chemicals that stir up inflammation and, as we have seen, digest enemies that have been "swallowed." Finally, the eosinophil's granules contain not only chemicals that modify allergic reactions and kill parasites but also potent toxins that contribute to certain rare diseases of the nervous system.

The neutrophil can also be assigned to a third category with which we are already familiar, the *nonspecific effector cells*. These are cells that are capable of destroying foreign invaders on first sight, without the prior programming required by B- and T-cells. Circulating macrophages are nonspecific effectors, as is another type of cell, the *natural killer*, or *NK*, *cell*. Some scientists consider the NK cell to be a relative of B- and T-cells. What *is* known is that it recognizes cancer and virus-infected cells by mechanisms different from those used by other immune cells and kills them without immune system assistance.

Other White Blood Cell Groups

Granulocytes

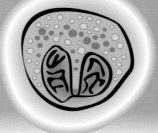

Eosinophil

The eosinophil's granules contain chemicals for the killing and digestion of parasites, a toxin that causes nervous system diseases, and other chemicals that work with and against the allergy-causing agents produced by the basophil. Eosinophil granules stain red on a microscope slide.

Phagocytes

The first step of phagocytosis involves adherence of the invading organism to the surface of the phagocyte.

The membrane of the phagocyte then wraps itself around the intruder.

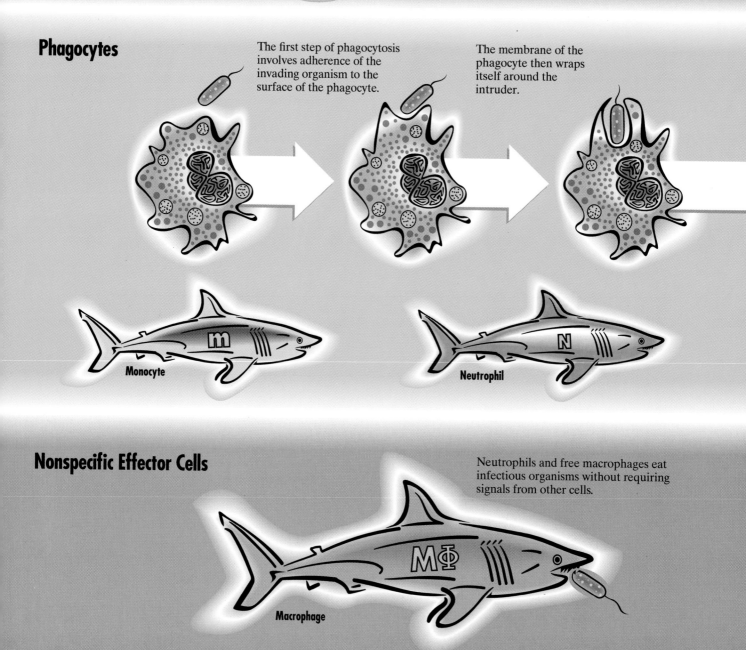

Monocyte

Neutrophil

Nonspecific Effector Cells

Neutrophils and free macrophages eat infectious organisms without requiring signals from other cells.

Macrophage

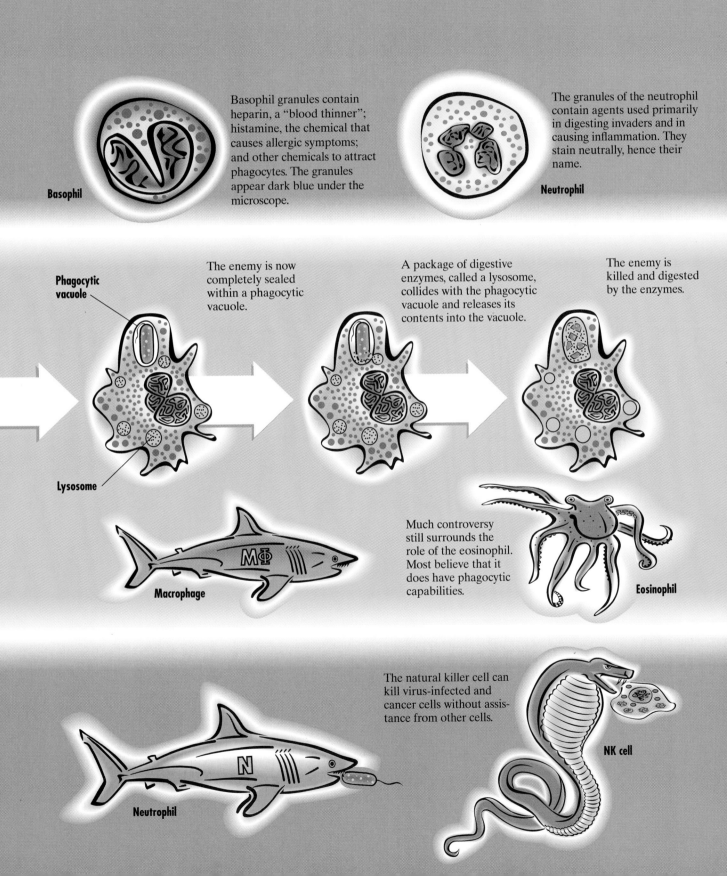

Basophil

Basophil granules contain heparin, a "blood thinner"; histamine, the chemical that causes allergic symptoms; and other chemicals to attract phagocytes. The granules appear dark blue under the microscope.

Neutrophil

The granules of the neutrophil contain agents used primarily in digesting invaders and in causing inflammation. They stain neutrally, hence their name.

Phagocytic vacuole

Lysosome

The enemy is now completely sealed within a phagocytic vacuole.

A package of digestive enzymes, called a lysosome, collides with the phagocytic vacuole and releases its contents into the vacuole.

The enemy is killed and digested by the enzymes.

Macrophage

Much controversy still surrounds the role of the eosinophil. Most believe that it does have phagocytic capabilities.

Eosinophil

The natural killer cell can kill virus-infected and cancer cells without assistance from other cells.

NK cell

Neutrophil

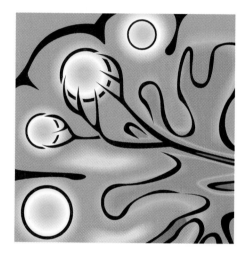

The Body's System of Filtration and Garbage Disposal

BLOOD IS NOT the only fluid that circulates throughout the body. Another important liquid, called *lymph*, squeezes between the cells that make up the organs of the body and cleanses them of infectious organisms, dead cells, and other particulate matter. Unlike blood, lymph's main function is to drain the tissues rather than to supply them with oxygen and nutrients. Lymph travels via *lymphatic vessels* to the various *lymphoid organs* (for example, lymph nodes, spleen, and tonsils), which filter the lymph of debris before it empties into the bloodstream. Because the lymphoid organs are areas where foreign invaders tend to collect, they are ideal sites for T- and B-cells to be exposed to the enemies that they will eventually combat.

T-cells from the thymus and B-cells from (presumably) the bone marrow are carried by the blood into the lymph node through a conduit called the *high endothelial* or *postcapillary venule*. The foreign intruder, called an *antigen* because it leads to the production of antibody, is carried by a monocyte or macrophage through another entrance, the *afferent lymphatic vessel*. The T-cell meets antigen in a part of the lymph node known as the *paracortex*, whereas the B-cell encounters antigen in the *germinal center*. B- and T-cells are activated by contact with antigens specific for their receptors and are thenceforth ready to defend the body against invasion by those antigens. They then exit the lymph node through *efferent lymphatic vessels*, which eventually empty into the bloodstream near the heart via the *thoracic* and *right lymphatic ducts*.

This *lymphatic system* is intimately linked with a collection of cells called the *reticuloendothelial system*, or *RES*, also known as the *mononuclear phagocyte system*, or *MPS*. We were introduced to this system in Chapters 1 and 2. The RES comprises monocytes and macrophages in the spleen, lymph nodes, liver, bone marrow, lungs, and lymphoid portions of the intestines called *Peyer's patches*. The cells of the RES are the "garbage collectors" of the body and are responsible for eating bacteria, old blood cells, and foreign particles polluting the blood. Some macrophages are confined to their specific organ, such as the *Kupffer cells* of the liver and the *alveolar macrophages* of the lung, and are adapted to thrive in these particular environments; other macrophages are free to circulate and hunt down the enemy (free macrophages).

We can use the spleen as an example of how this disposal system works. Blood enters the spleen through the *splenic artery*, which divides into progressively smaller branches. The smallest branches, called *central arteries*, pass through the *white pulp* of the spleen and into the *red pulp*, which is packed with thin cords that are lined with hungry macrophages. The blood is cleared of any foreign matter and then empties into *venous sinuses*, which converge to form the outgoing *splenic vein*.

We are now familiar with all the components of the immune system and how they work. Next we will take what we've learned and examine how the immune system is involved in various disease processes. Chapters 11 and 12 will cover one such topic that is familiar to us all—allergies.

The Reticuloendothelial and Lymphatic Systems

The reticuloendothelial and lymphatic systems serve two important functions. They clear the blood and tissues of foreign debris, and they provide sites where immune system cells can be activated.

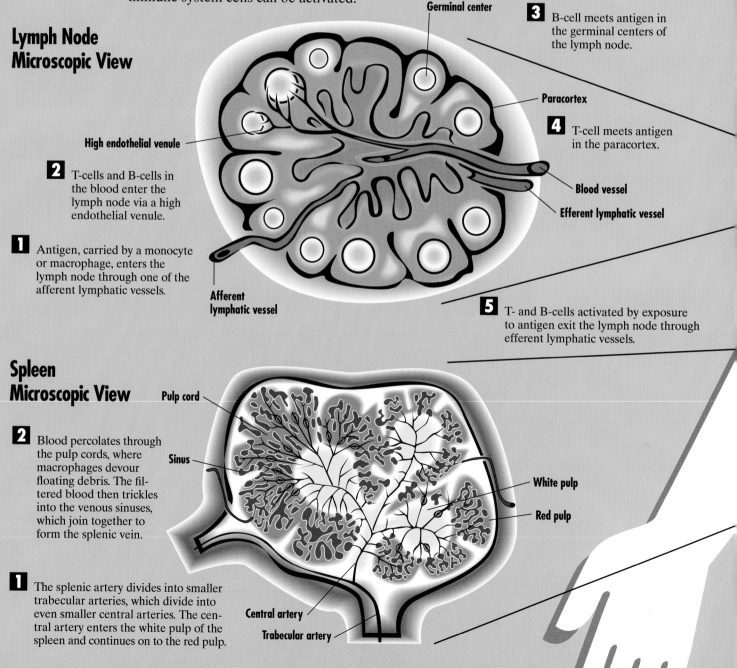

Lymph Node Microscopic View

2 T-cells and B-cells in the blood enter the lymph node via a high endothelial venule.

1 Antigen, carried by a monocyte or macrophage, enters the lymph node through one of the afferent lymphatic vessels.

High endothelial venule

Afferent lymphatic vessel

Germinal center

3 B-cell meets antigen in the germinal centers of the lymph node.

Paracortex

4 T-cell meets antigen in the paracortex.

Blood vessel

Efferent lymphatic vessel

5 T- and B-cells activated by exposure to antigen exit the lymph node through efferent lymphatic vessels.

Spleen Microscopic View

2 Blood percolates through the pulp cords, where macrophages devour floating debris. The filtered blood then trickles into the venous sinuses, which join together to form the splenic vein.

1 The splenic artery divides into smaller trabecular arteries, which divide into even smaller central arteries. The central artery enters the white pulp of the spleen and continues on to the red pulp.

Pulp cord

Sinus

White pulp

Red pulp

Central artery

Trabecular artery

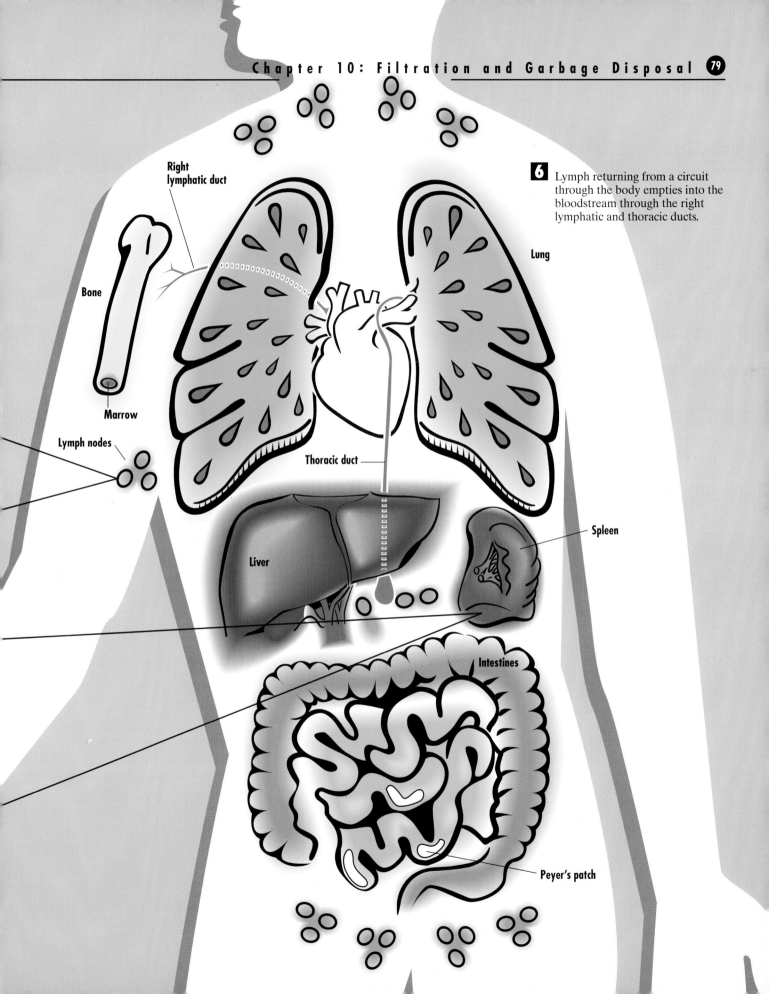

Right lymphatic duct

Bone

Marrow

Lymph nodes

6 Lymph returning from a circuit through the body empties into the bloodstream through the right lymphatic and thoracic ducts.

Lung

Thoracic duct

Liver

Spleen

Intestines

Peyer's patch

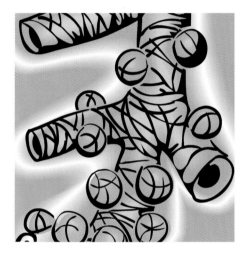

Allergies, Asthma, and Anaphylaxis

AN *ALLERGY* IS an overreaction of the body's immune system to what is ordinarily a harmless foreign substance. As we saw in Chapter 7, a specific type of antibody, called *IgE*, is active primarily in allergic reactions and parasitic infections. Many scientists believe that the allergies of today stem from ancestral antiparasitic defenses. Because so few people in industrialized societies encounter parasites on a routine basis, the IgE that originally protected our ancestors from these organisms now devotes itself to allergic reactions.

For a person to become allergic to a substance, the immune system must first undergo a process called *sensitization*, which can take place on the initial exposure to the offending agent or at a later date. Sensitization is a concept that is not fully understood, and a means of identifying those people who will eventually develop an allergy has yet to be discovered. What is known is that allergy-prone people tend to have higher blood levels of IgE antibody than nonallergic people. Some researchers think this may be the result of DNA enhancing the production of IgE, at the expense of IgM and IgG, in response to certain antigens. This genetic explanation makes sense because allergic tendencies can be inherited. Another theory postulates that people with allergies may be less able to control histamine release from basophils and mast cells than nonallergic people. Obviously, the mere presence of elevated IgE levels allows more basophils and mast cells to be stimulated into releasing their contents.

Sensitization occurs when an *allergen* like pollen, dust, or insect venom enters the body and is consumed by macrophages. The macrophage breaks the allergen into pieces and displays them on its surface, where the helper T-cell can "see" them. Once the T-cell recognizes the allergen, it signals the B-cell to transform into a plasma cell and begin secreting IgE antibody. The IgE molecules then attach to the surfaces of *mast cells* within the tissues of the body or *basophils* in the blood. The sensitization process is complete at this point, but no symptoms have occurred—sensitization merely primes the immune system for a rapid response against future invasions by the same allergen. Therefore, any adverse reaction to a substance on the very first exposure is *not* an allergic response.

When an allergen enters the body of a sensitized person, it binds to the IgE molecules that stud the basophil and mast cell surfaces. The basophil/mast cell becomes activated when an allergen binds two IgEs simultaneously, thus *cross-linking* them. The basophil/mast cell then releases *histamine* and other chemicals that cause mucus production, breathing difficulty, sneezing, itching, swelling, redness, and all the other symptoms commonly associated with allergic reactions. Histamine can also draw other immune cells, like eosinophils and monocytes, into the site of the allergic reaction, where they can cause long-term inflammation and other symptoms.

Allergic reactions take different forms in different people. The most common form is *seasonal allergic rhinitis*, or *hayfever*, which is elicited by the pollen and spores released from trees, grasses, and weeds during certain times of the year. Other people suffer *perennial allergic rhinitis*, a year-round hypersensitivity to dust mites and other indoor allergens. In some individuals, allergic reactions are so intense that they lead to *extrinsic asthma*, a condition characterized by wheezing and shortness of breath from inflammation and constriction of the airways. *Intrinsic asthma* shares these symptoms but is not associated with allergies.

A minority of allergy sufferers react to allergens in the worst possible way. *Anaphylaxis* is a rapid allergic reaction that results from an explosive release by mast cells and basophils, causing airway closure and blood vessel dilatation, which, in the absence of treatment, ultimately lead to shock and death. Prompt injection of *epinephrine* brings about a rapid reversal of symptoms.

Treatment of the other types of allergic reactions depends on the severity of the symptoms. For most, *antihistamines*, which, as their name implies, block the effects of histamine, suffice. People with asthmatic symptoms often obtain relief through the use of *bronchodilator* pills or inhalers, which relax tightened airways. Those with more serious problems may require *adrenocorticosteroids*, which are synthetic versions of potent antiinflammatory hormones produced by the *adrenal gland*. Others may benefit from regular *extract injections*, in which increasingly larger doses of an allergen are given in an attempt to desensitize. There are nearly as many ways to treat allergies as there are allergy sufferers, and each treatment regimen must be tailored to the individual.

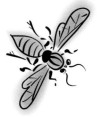

Sensitization and Histamine Release

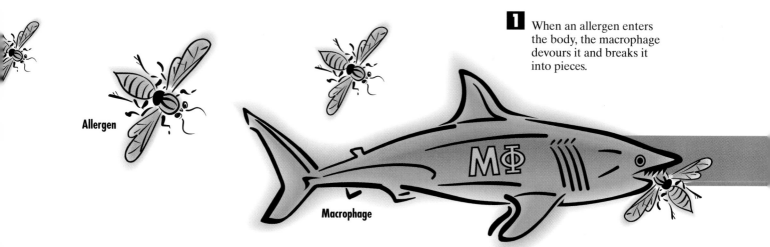

1 When an allergen enters the body, the macrophage devours it and breaks it into pieces.

Allergen

Macrophage

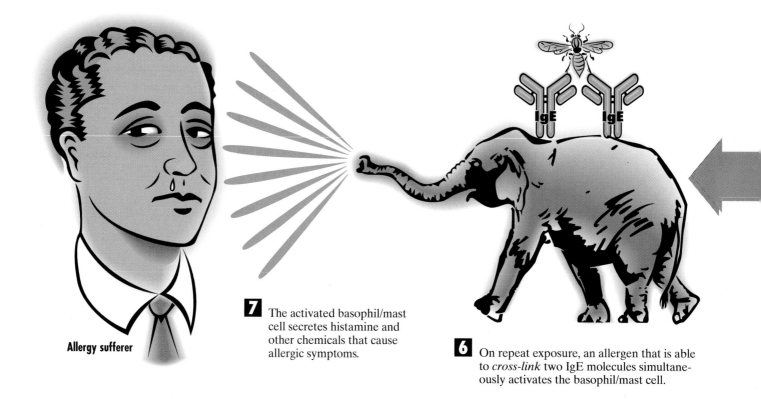

Allergy sufferer

7 The activated basophil/mast cell secretes histamine and other chemicals that cause allergic symptoms.

IgE **IgE**

6 On repeat exposure, an allergen that is able to *cross-link* two IgE molecules simultaneously activates the basophil/mast cell.

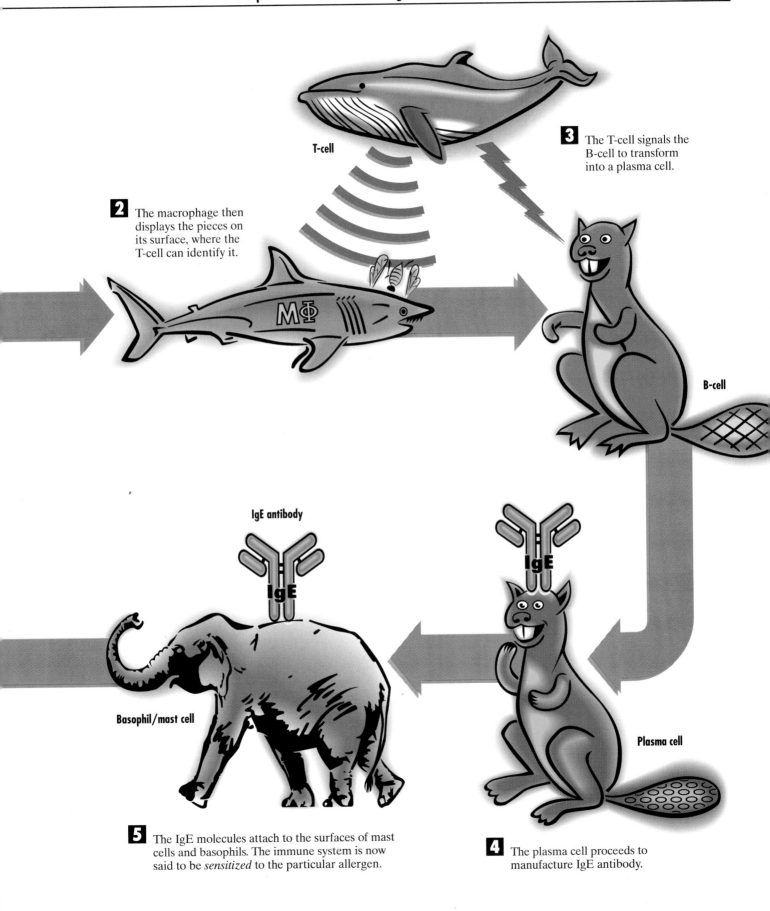

T-cell

3 The T-cell signals the B-cell to transform into a plasma cell.

2 The macrophage then displays the pieces on its surface, where the T-cell can identify it.

B-cell

IgE antibody

IgE

Basophil/mast cell

Plasma cell

5 The IgE molecules attach to the surfaces of mast cells and basophils. The immune system is now said to be *sensitized* to the particular allergen.

4 The plasma cell proceeds to manufacture IgE antibody.

Asthma and Anaphylaxis

Asthma

Asthma is characterized by inflammation and swelling of the inner surface of the *bronchi*, or airways, with excessive production of mucus, which can actually obstruct airflow.

Obstruction of normal breathing is further exacerbated by contraction of the *smooth muscle* encircling the bronchioles, which are small bronchi (airways).

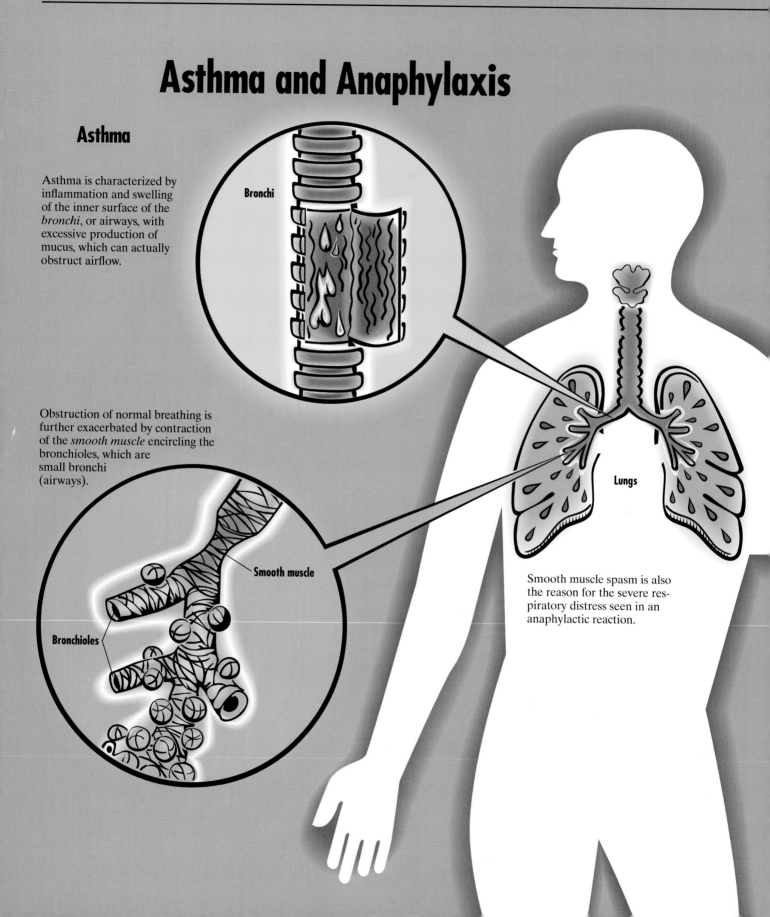

Bronchi

Smooth muscle

Bronchioles

Lungs

Smooth muscle spasm is also the reason for the severe respiratory distress seen in an anaphylactic reaction.

Anaphylaxis

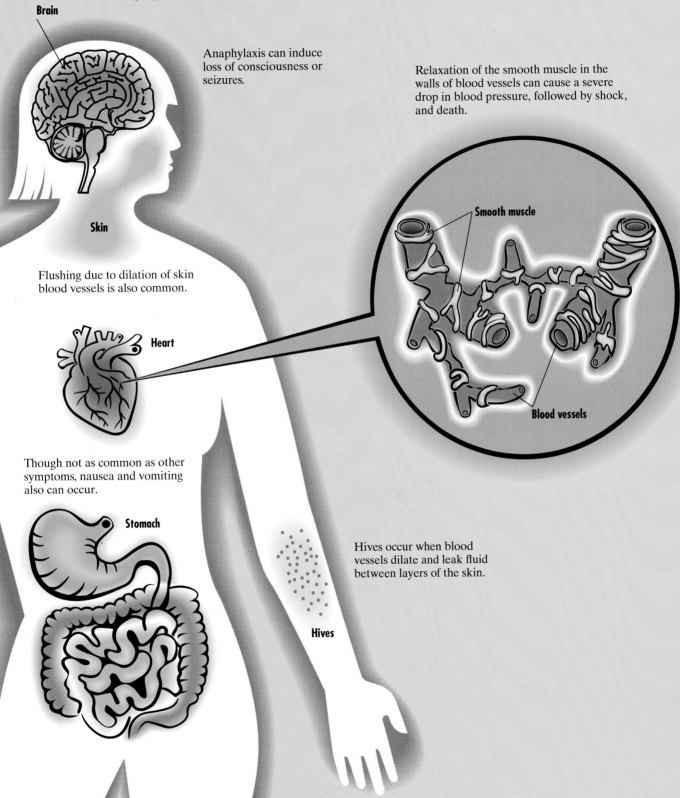

Brain

Anaphylaxis can induce loss of consciousness or seizures.

Relaxation of the smooth muscle in the walls of blood vessels can cause a severe drop in blood pressure, followed by shock, and death.

Skin

Flushing due to dilation of skin blood vessels is also common.

Smooth muscle

Heart

Blood vessels

Though not as common as other symptoms, nausea and vomiting also can occur.

Stomach

Hives occur when blood vessels dilate and leak fluid between layers of the skin.

Hives

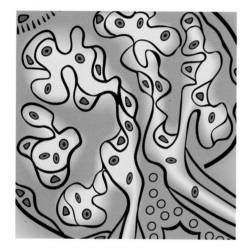

Other Hypersensitivities

THE ALLERGIES DEALT with in the previous chapter were *type I,* or *immediate type, hypersensitivity* reactions, meaning that they result from histamine release following contact with an allergen. The three other types of hypersensitivity reactions are covered in this chapter. They all have in common an overreaction by the immune system to an antigen, resulting in symptoms.

A *type II hypersensitivity* reaction occurs when antibody or complement attaches to a person's own cells or tissues. For example, blood types are designated as A, B, AB, or O, depending upon which antigens and antibodies are present. There are some other, more obscure, blood groups that health care personnel also use to ensure that transfused blood will be accepted by the recipient's immune system. However, a person sometimes receives donated blood that is regarded as foreign by the immune system, leading to the attachment of antibody to the donor's red blood cells and their subsequent destruction. This is a *transfusion incompatibility* reaction, a form of type II hypersensitivity.

Classic examples of type II hypersensitivity are the *immunohemolytic anemias*, also called *Coombs-positive* hemolytic anemias because they exhibit positive *Coombs tests* for antibodies that attack red blood cells. In these disorders, anemia results from the destruction of red blood cells that have been tagged for termination by antibodies. Immunohemolytic anemias are seen in a variety of diseases, including Hodgkin's lymphoma and chronic leukemia, or as the result of certain infections or drug reactions.

Symptoms associated with the immunohemolytic anemias vary, depending on the type. Those caused by "warm" antibodies, which are active at normal body temperature, are characterized by weakness, jaundice, and enlargement of the spleen and liver. Stiff, blue fingers and toes following exposure to low temperatures are common features of the "cold" antibody immunohemolytic anemias. Treatment for the "warm" type ranges from high-dose *adrenocorticosteroids* (steroids, for short) to removal of the spleen, whereas avoidance of cold usually suffices for the other type.

Another important type II hypersensitivity reaction is the *hyperacute rejection* of transplanted organs. This is the destruction of a donor organ in a matter of minutes or hours, because the recipient's immune system has been previously exposed to antigens contained in the organ. This *presensitization* can occur as the result of a transfusion, pregnancy, or prior transplantation. Other type II hypersensitivity syndromes exist.

Usually, when invasion by an antigen causes the production of antibody, the two bind together into an *antigen-antibody complex* that is consumed by macrophages. Sometimes, however, as in the case of lupus, rheumatoid arthritis, or certain kidney diseases, the complexes deposit into tissues and small blood vessels, where they stimulate the immune system into wreaking havoc. This is a *type III hypersensitivity* reaction. The immune complexes activate complement, which attracts neutrophils and monocytes to the scene. These cells then release their digestive chemicals, causing inflammation and tissue damage.

The archetypal type III hypersensitivity reaction is *serum sickness*, which can occur after the administration of penicillin or one of the horse-serum antitoxins. One to two weeks after such a medication is given, circulating antigen-antibody complexes cause fever, malaise, skin eruptions, joint pain, depressed white blood cell count, enlarged lymph nodes, and urinary protein excretion. The treatment for this and other type III reactions is to remove the offending substance and suppress the inflammation. For more severe reactions, steroids may be required.

The final type of hypersensitivity reaction is familiar to anyone who has ever had a rash from poison ivy, oak, or sumac. This is the *type IV*, or *delayed-type, hypersensitivity* (DTH) reaction. Unlike the other three hypersensitivities, this type is caused by sensitized T-cells rather than by antibody. After an initial exposure to a particular antigen, memory T-cells persist for anywhere from days to years until a subsequent exposure to the same antigen causes them to multiply. The T-cell clones signal inflammatory cells, such as macrophages and neutrophils, to the area, where chemicals are released that result in tissue injury.

Contact dermatitis is undoubtedly the most common DTH reaction. Direct contact with a plant, such as poison ivy, or with a number of other substances, such as topical medications, fabrics, metals, dyes, or cosmetics, leads to the widely recognized rash and blisters that characterize this dermatologic condition. A positive TB skin test in a person previously exposed to this bacterium is another example of a DTH reaction. In addition, most cases of *transplant rejection* are the result of sensitized T-cells attacking donor organs, and they are therefore classified as type IV hypersensitivities. This topic will be covered in greater detail in Chapter 16.

Type II Hypersensitivity

Blood Type Compatibility

Type A blood has type A antigen on the red blood cells and antibody against type B blood (anti-B) in the serum. A transfusion with type B or AB blood leads to an incompatibility reaction.

Type B blood has type B antigen on the red blood cells and anti-A antibody in the serum. Types A and AB are incompatible.

Type AB blood has A and B antigens, but no antibodies, so a person with type AB blood can receive transfusions of any blood type. For this reason, type AB blood is called the universal recipient.

Type O blood has anti-A and anti-B antibodies, but no antigens, so anyone can receive a transfusion with type O blood. Thus, type O blood is designated as the universal donor.

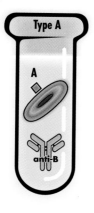

Type A

A

anti-B

Type B

B

anti-A

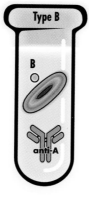

Type AB

A B

Type O

anti-A

anti-B

Many other blood type antigens exist and must be matched as closely as possible between donor and recipient in order to avoid incompatibility reactions. Rh (positive or negative) is the most important of these other blood groups, but Kell, Duffy, Lutheran, and others are also important.

Red blood cell

Hyperacute Transplant Rejection

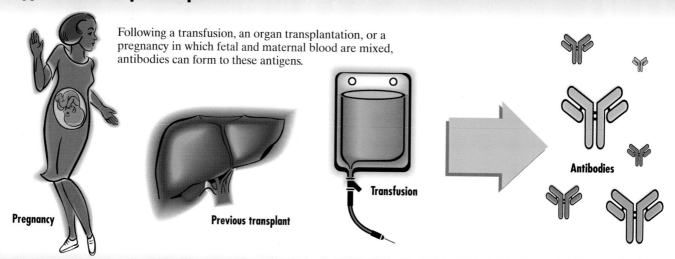

Following a transfusion, an organ transplantation, or a pregnancy in which fetal and maternal blood are mixed, antibodies can form to these antigens.

Antibodies

Transfusion

Pregnancy

Previous transplant

Immunohemolytic Anemias

"Cold" antibodies against red blood cells can form following mononucleosis or "walking" pneumonia infections and are usually of the IgM type.

"Warm" antibodies against red blood cells can occur in the setting of lupus, lymphoma, or leukemia, and they are usually of the IgG type.

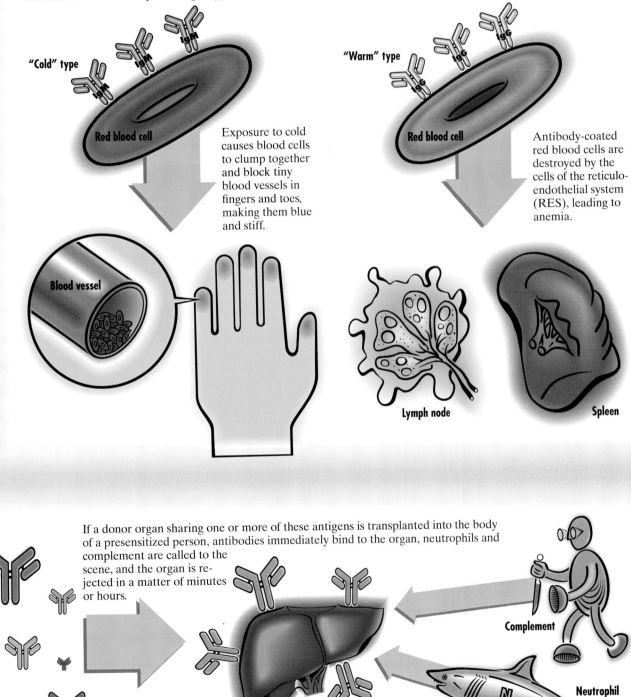

"Cold" type

Red blood cell

Exposure to cold causes blood cells to clump together and block tiny blood vessels in fingers and toes, making them blue and stiff.

Blood vessel

"Warm" type

Red blood cell

Antibody-coated red blood cells are destroyed by the cells of the reticulo-endothelial system (RES), leading to anemia.

Lymph node

Spleen

If a donor organ sharing one or more of these antigens is transplanted into the body of a presensitized person, antibodies immediately bind to the organ, neutrophils and complement are called to the scene, and the organ is rejected in a matter of minutes or hours.

Complement

Neutrophil

Donor organ

Types III and IV Hypersensitivities

Type III Hypersensitivity

In serum sickness, the classic type III hypersensitivity reaction, an antigen such as penicillin enters the body and leads to the production of antibodies, usually of the IgG type.

The antigen and antibody join together as an antigen-antibody complex.

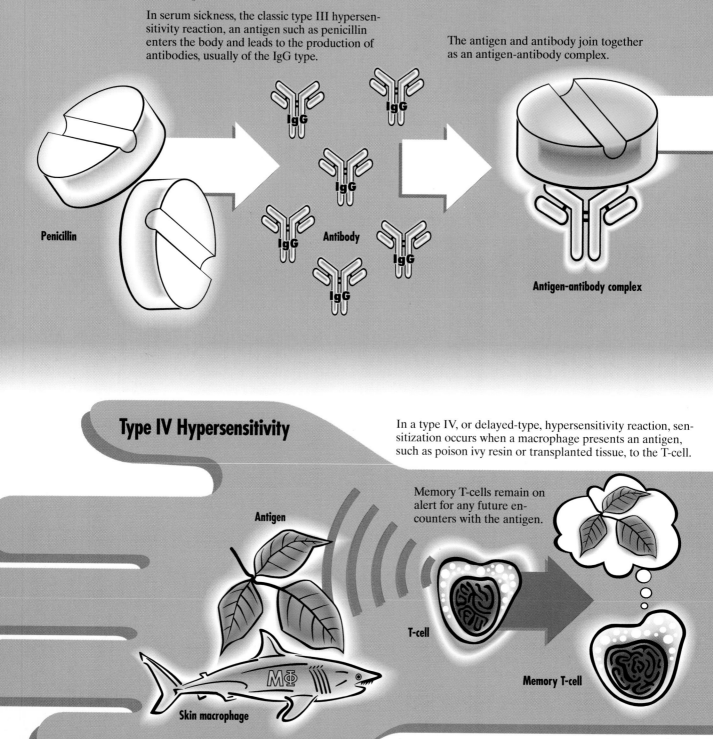

Penicillin

IgG IgG IgG IgG IgG IgG

Antibody

Antigen-antibody complex

Type IV Hypersensitivity

In a type IV, or delayed-type, hypersensitivity reaction, sensitization occurs when a macrophage presents an antigen, such as poison ivy resin or transplanted tissue, to the T-cell.

Memory T-cells remain on alert for any future encounters with the antigen.

Antigen

T-cell

Memory T-cell

Skin macrophage

The antigen-antibody complexes circulate and deposit in the microscopic blood vessels of the kidney and other organs. Here they attract inflammatory cells, which secrete chemicals that damage the organ. A similar form of kidney damage is seen in lupus.

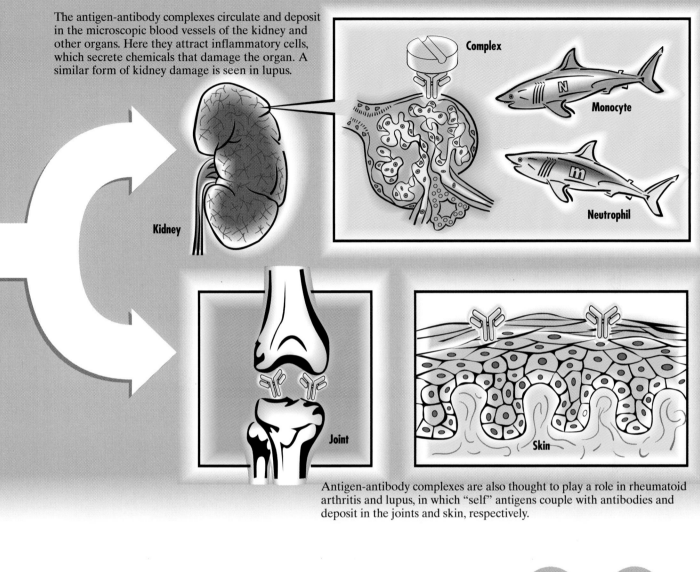

Antigen-antibody complexes are also thought to play a role in rheumatoid arthritis and lupus, in which "self" antigens couple with antibodies and deposit in the joints and skin, respectively.

A subsequent exposure causes the T-cell to secrete chemicals that attract inflammatory cells to the scene.

In the case of poison ivy, inflammatory cells create the characteristic rash and blisters.

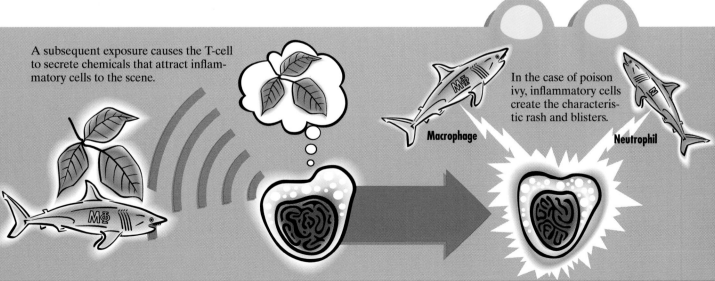

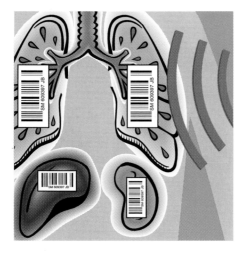

CHAPTER 13

How the Body Distinguishes "Self" from "Non-self"

I N CHAPTER 1, we briefly touched on the concept of "self" versus "non-self." The term "self" is applied to any organ that is identified by the immune system as native tissue and is left alone, while "non-self" tissue is regarded as foreign and is attacked. The classic example of non-self tissue eliciting an immune response is the transplantation of a donor organ into another body. The recipient's immune system immediately recognizes it as foreign and rejects it.

The immune system's primary means of differentiating "self" from "non-self" is the *human leukocyte group A*, or *HLA*. This group of antigens, found on almost every cell in the body, is determined by a particular segment of our DNA called the *major histocompatibility complex (MHC)*, which we already know to be the selector of T-cell types and the manufacturer of the transport molecules that move infectious organisms to the surfaces of cells. In fact, the MHC transport molecules with which we are familiar are examples of HLA antigens. You can think of the HLA as being the body's "serial number." The immune system recognizes a transplanted organ as foreign mainly on the basis of its unfamiliar HLA. The closer the HLAs of the donor and the recipient can be matched, the greater the likelihood that the transplanted organ will survive.

How do our immune system cells develop this ability to recognize self organs and reject non-self organs? In Chapter 6, we saw that the ability of B-cells to make millions of different antibodies derives from our inheritance of antibody-making "machinery" in parts that can be reassembled in many different ways. We then learned how abnormal and self-reactive B-cells are destroyed before they reach the circulation. These two concepts also apply to T-cells.

The segments of DNA responsible for manufacturing the receptors that T-cells use to identify foreign invaders are inherited as pieces that can be combined in over 100 million different ways. This allows each T-cell to be specific for only one particular antigen presented by one particular MHC molecule. However, having so many ways of assembling T-cell receptors inevitably leads to the construction of T-cells that are incapable of functioning properly or that have receptors which recognize normal body structures. In order to maintain healthy immune function, such cells are eliminated.

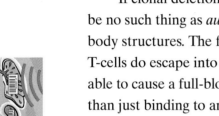

The *clonal deletion theory* is the most widely accepted explanation of how the body disposes of undesirable T-cells. While humans are in the embryonic stages of development, antigens are presented to immature T-cells in the thymus. As we saw in Chapter 8, those cells presented with antigen by *class I MHC* molecules eventually become *killer* or *suppressor* T-cells, whereas those receiving antigen from *class II MHC* become *helper* or *inflammatory* T-cells. T-cells which bind neither type of MHC die before reaching maturity. Those which bind "self" antigen (self-reactive T-cells) that is presented by MHC are quickly destroyed. The remaining T-cells are those which bind MHC but not "self" antigen, and they are allowed to mature. Activation of these normal T-cells occurs later, when foreign antigen is presented to them by the appropriate MHC.

If clonal deletion ensured the destruction of all self-reactive T-cells, there would be no such thing as *autoimmune diseases,* in which immune system cells attack normal body structures. The fact that such diseases exist must mean that some self-reactive T-cells do escape into the circulation. However, most mature self-reactive cells are not able to cause a full-blown autoimmune disease. The reason is that a T-cell requires more than just binding to an antigen in order to exert its effects. It relies on an additional signal, usually from a B-cell or macrophage, before it can act. Self-reactive T-cells that do not receive this crucial signal are summarily destroyed.

Self-Recognition

Every person has a unique group of antigens, called the HLA, that is present on almost every cell in the body. The HLA is the "serial number" that the immune system uses to distinguish "self" organs from "non-self" organs.

The immune system recognizes donor organs as "non-self" primarily on the basis of their unfamiliar HLA.

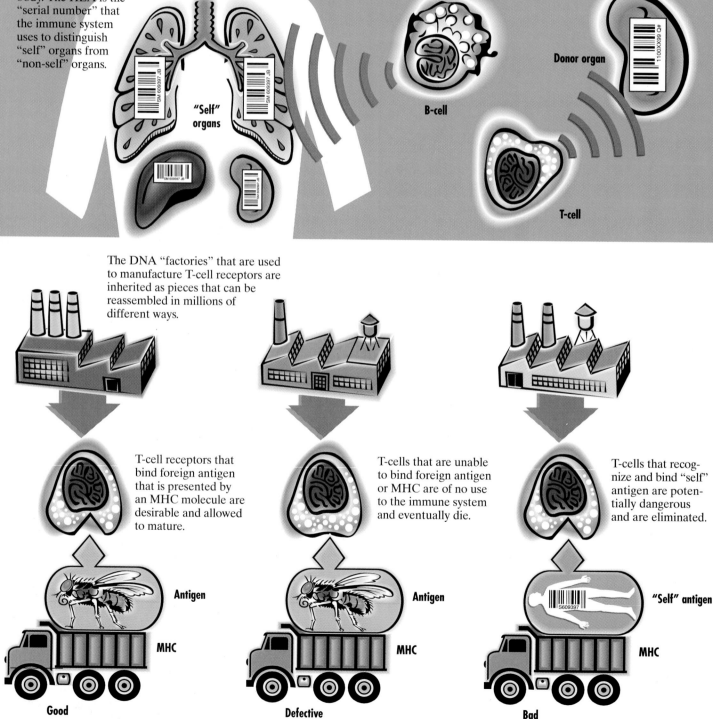

"Self" organs

B-cell

Donor organ

T-cell

The DNA "factories" that are used to manufacture T-cell receptors are inherited as pieces that can be reassembled in millions of different ways.

T-cell receptors that bind foreign antigen that is presented by an MHC molecule are desirable and allowed to mature.

T-cells that are unable to bind foreign antigen or MHC are of no use to the immune system and eventually die.

T-cells that recognize and bind "self" antigen are potentially dangerous and are eliminated.

Antigen

MHC

Good

Antigen

MHC

Defective

"Self" antigen

MHC

Bad

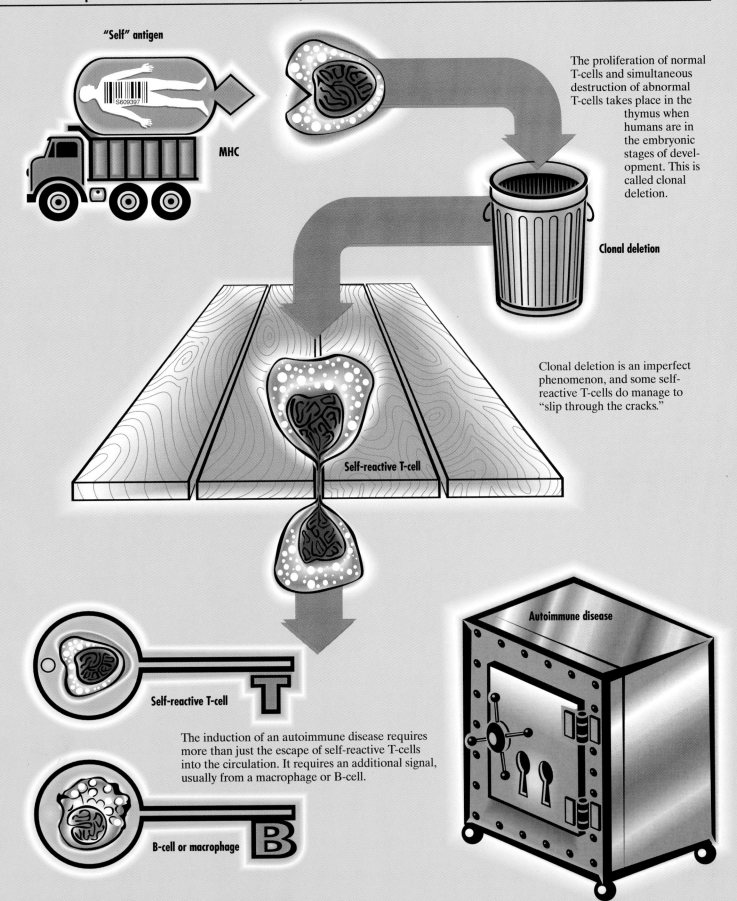

"Self" antigen

MHC

The proliferation of normal T-cells and simultaneous destruction of abnormal T-cells takes place in the thymus when humans are in the embryonic stages of development. This is called clonal deletion.

Clonal deletion

Clonal deletion is an imperfect phenomenon, and some self-reactive T-cells do manage to "slip through the cracks."

Self-reactive T-cell

Self-reactive T-cell

B-cell or macrophage

The induction of an autoimmune disease requires more than just the escape of self-reactive T-cells into the circulation. It requires an additional signal, usually from a macrophage or B-cell.

Autoimmune disease

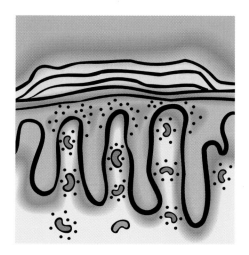

Autoimmune Diseases

T-CELLS THAT ESCAPE into the circulation, bind with "self" antigen, and receive appropriate signals from macrophages or B-cells can eventually lead to the development of *autoimmune diseases*. These are disorders in which a person's immune system confuses normal body tissue with foreign antigen and attacks it. There are several proposed mechanisms by which these cases of mistaken identity evolve.

One explanation stems from the fact that many autoimmune diseases follow a bacterial or viral infection. As a way of avoiding an attack by the immune system, certain infectious organisms learn to expose only those parts of themselves that the immune system will recognize as "self" antigens. When the immune system does mount a response against these organisms, it inadvertently targets the "self" organs that the enemy has attempted to imitate. This is an example of a *cross-reaction*, in which an immune system that is primed to respond to one antigen also responds to a similar antigen, and this process is called *molecular mimicry*. Genetics play a significant role in deciding whether molecular mimicry will lead to a full-blown autoimmune disease. It is the HLA, the body's "serial number," that determines which part of an infectious organism will be presented to the cells of the immune system. As a result of this genetic factor, the tendency to develop an autoimmune disease can be inherited.

The molecular mimicry model may help explain how a number of autoimmune diseases occur. For example, portions of a particular virus, called adenovirus type 2, look remarkably similar to the materials that compose the *myelin sheath*, which is the protective covering that surrounds nerves and parts of the brain. When the immune system attacks this virus, it can also mistakenly attack the myelin sheath and cause *multiple sclerosis (MS)*. Similarly, in fighting off certain streptococcal bacteria, the immune system may also target valves of the heart, leading to *rheumatic fever*. A defense against tuberculosis may expand to include the cartilage lining certain joints and result in *rheumatoid arthritis (RA)*. Several viruses have been implicated as possible molecular mimics in the development of *diabetes mellitus*.

A second mechanism for acquiring an autoimmune disease could be a release into the circulation of antigens that normally are hidden from the immune system. When these sequestered antigens escape by traumatic or other means, the immune system regards them as "non-self" and attacks them. This mechanism may explain the occurrence of certain autoimmune diseases of the eye, heart, and male reproductive system.

Third, "self" antigens can be altered by an infection, a chemical, or ultraviolet radiation and take on the appearance of "non-self" antigens. Fourth, some cases of lymphoma may be the result of mutations in immune system cells, which lead to the secretion of antibodies against "self" structures, rather than the result of antigen mutations. Finally, a defect in the function of *suppressor T-cells*, which are designed to keep potentially self-reactive T-cells under control, may also play a role in autoimmune diseases.

In order for self-reactive T-cells to cause an autoimmune disease, they must escape from the circulation and travel to their target organ. The first step in accomplishing this task is the secretion of chemicals by T-cells and macrophages that cause the linings of blood vessels to become "sticky." Circulating T-cells that would otherwise float past the target organ thus adhere to the walls of blood vessels and begin boring holes in them using digestive chemicals. The T-cells then squeeze through the holes to reach their destination, where the HLA presents "self" antigen to them. The T-cells respond by secreting chemicals that cause tissue damage and by attracting macrophages, which compound the damage by eating away at body tissue and secreting chemicals of their own.

Virtually any organ of the body can be the target of an autoimmune process. As we have seen, the myelin sheath and the linings of joints are attacked in MS and RA, respectively. Many scientists believe that the destruction of insulin-producing cells of the pancreas by self-reactive immune system cells is a major cause of *diabetes mellitus*. In *myasthenia gravis*, the connections between nerves and muscles are affected. In *Graves' disease*, immune system cells cause the thyroid gland to secrete excessive amounts of thyroid hormone. Skin is targeted in *pemphigus vulgaris* and *psoriasis*. An unidentified antigen leads to the development of *sarcoidosis*, a disease in which focal areas of inflammation, called *granulomas*, appear in multiple organs, including the lungs, liver, heart, eyes, and skin.

Systemic lupus erythematosus (SLE), or *lupus*, is an inflammatory disorder of the *connective tissue*, which is the fibrous, elastic, fatty, or cartilaginous matrix that connects and supports other tissues. Connective tissue is found in almost every organ; therefore, the manifestations of lupus affect almost every organ system, including eyes, blood vessels, intestinal tract, kidneys, heart, lungs, brain and nerves, blood, skin, muscle, and bone. In addition to being an autoimmune disease, lupus also has features of type II and type III hypersensitivities. *Antinuclear antibodies (ANA)* form against "self" structures (type II), and antigen-antibody complexes deposit in microscopic blood vessels (type III). The choice of treatment for lupus depends on the severity of symptoms. Mild cases usually respond to antiinflammatory drugs, whereas people with more severe illnesses may require steroids or chemotherapeutic drugs. However, none of these treatment modalities is a cure for lupus.

Similarly, treatment for the other autoimmune diseases is usually aimed at lessening the severity of symptoms, rather than halting the disease process at its source. Oral sugar-lowering drugs are used in type II diabetes, while insulin injections are required for type I diabetes. RA is typically treated with nonsteroidal anti-inflammatory drugs or steroids; people with severe disabilities may require immunosuppressive drugs or surgery. Removal of the thymus alleviates the symptoms of myasthenia gravis. Depending on the age of the person, radioactive iodine or thyroid removal is used to treat Graves' disease. Steroids can sometimes improve the symptoms of MS, but no form of treatment is consistently effective in this disease.

Approximately half of all persons afflicted with an autoimmune disease experience periods of spontaneous remission and exacerbation, as opposed to a continuous worsening of symptoms. These cyclic variations appear to be related to some external factors. For example, excessive emotional stress in a person with MS can cause the brain to enhance the presentation of "self" antigen to T-cells by the HLA. The presence of female hormones can lead to similar results, which may explain why women tend to be more severely affected by autoimmune disorders than men. Finally, an infectious organism that invades the body of someone with an autoimmune disease can act as a "superantigen" in activating more self-reactive T-cells.

A great deal of research is currently directed toward finding more efficacious and specific treatment regimens for autoimmune diseases. Being able to rid the body of self-reactive T-cells is of particular interest. Oral doses of myelin may be able to stimulate helpful T-cells into counteracting the effects of harmful T-cells in MS. A protein called *beta interferon*, which is secreted by body cells as an antiviral defense, may be able to block the HLA and prevent it from being "read" by T-cells. Antibodies that prevent T-cells from "sticking" to target organ blood vessels may also be available some day. Research into antibodies against the genetic code that creates self-reactive receptors on T-cells also shows promise.

Causes of Autoimmune Diseases

Molecular Mimicry

Some infectious organisms display only those parts of themselves that resemble "self" antigen to the cells of the immune system in order to avoid triggering a response.

T-cell

When the immune system decides to mount a defense against the invading organism, it mistakenly targets the organ the intruder was attempting to mimic.

Infectious organism

The HLA is the body's "serial number" and is responsible for deciding which parts of an infectious organism are presented to immune system cells. The HLA is genetically determined, which explains why the tendency to develop an autoimmune disease can be inherited.

Macrophage

"Self" antigen

HLA

Altered "Self" Antigen

Sun

In people who are photosensitive, exposure to ultraviolet rays from the sun can alter proteins in the skin, causing them to resemble foreign antigen.

Red blood cell

Drug

Certain medications and chemicals can alter "self" antigen. For example, the blood pressure drug methyldopa can react chemically with the surfaces of red blood cells and cause them to appear foreign to the immune system. The immune system responds by producing antibodies that tag the "self" cells for destruction.

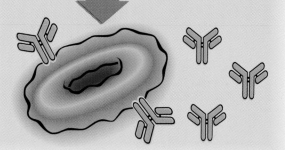

Mutation of Immune System Cells

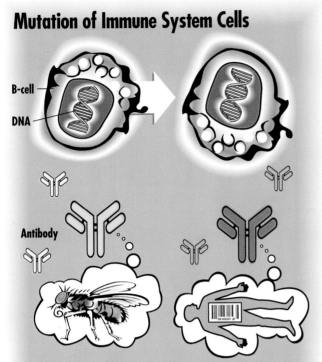

B-cell

DNA

Antibody

B-cells that produce normal antibody can mutate into cells that produce antibody against "self" organs. Such is the case in some forms of lymphoma.

Suppressor T-cell Defect

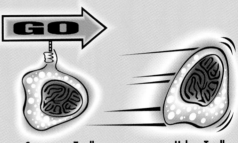

Helper T-cell

Suppressor T-cell

Suppressor T-cells, which normally moderate the activity of helper T-cells, can malfunction in certain autoimmune diseases.

GO

Suppressor T-cell

Helper T-cell

Release of Sequestered Antigen

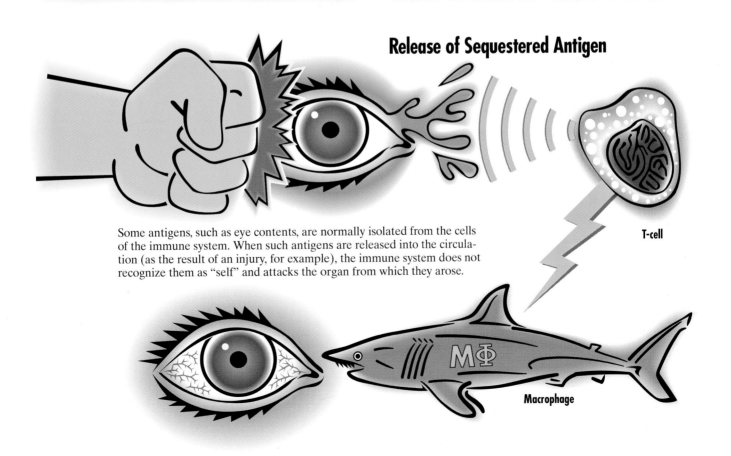

T-cell

Some antigens, such as eye contents, are normally isolated from the cells of the immune system. When such antigens are released into the circulation (as the result of an injury, for example), the immune system does not recognize them as "self" and attacks the organ from which they arose.

Macrophage

Tissue Damage in Autoimmune Diseases

In the absence of contributing factors, self-reactive T-cells would, like other blood cells, float past their intended target without causing damage.

Chemicals, called cytokines, are secreted by macrophages and T- cells at the target location and cause the blood vessel lining to become "sticky."

Macrophage

Blood vessel

T-cells

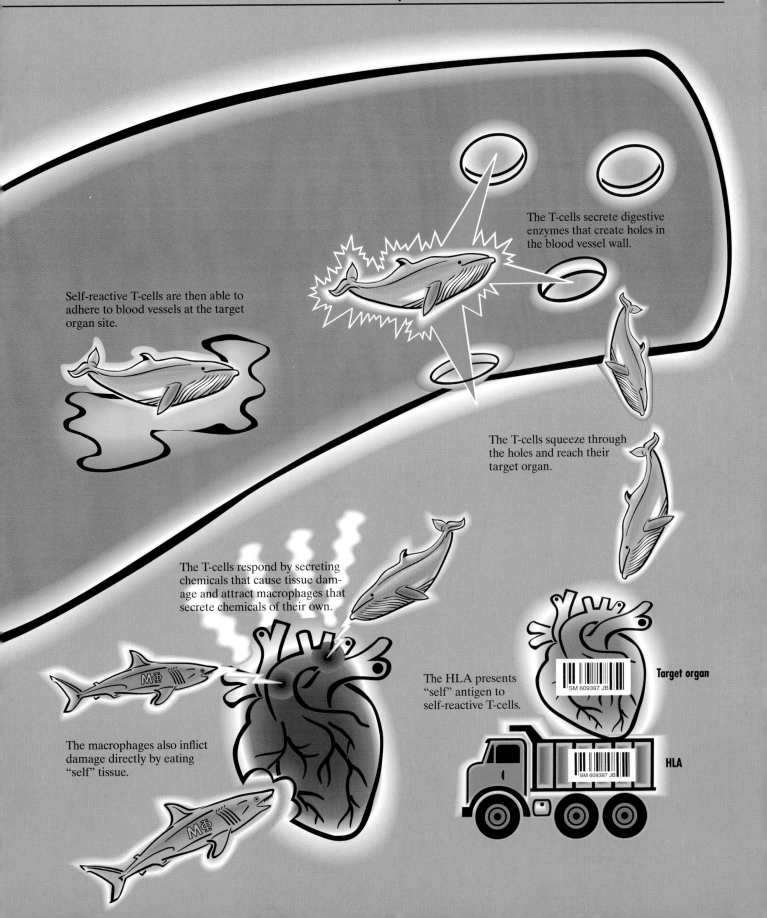

The T-cells secrete digestive enzymes that create holes in the blood vessel wall.

Self-reactive T-cells are then able to adhere to blood vessels at the target organ site.

The T-cells squeeze through the holes and reach their target organ.

The T-cells respond by secreting chemicals that cause tissue damage and attract macrophages that secrete chemicals of their own.

The HLA presents "self" antigen to self-reactive T-cells.

The macrophages also inflict damage directly by eating "self" tissue.

Target organ

HLA

SM 609397 JB

SM 609397 JB

Examples of Autoimmune Diseases

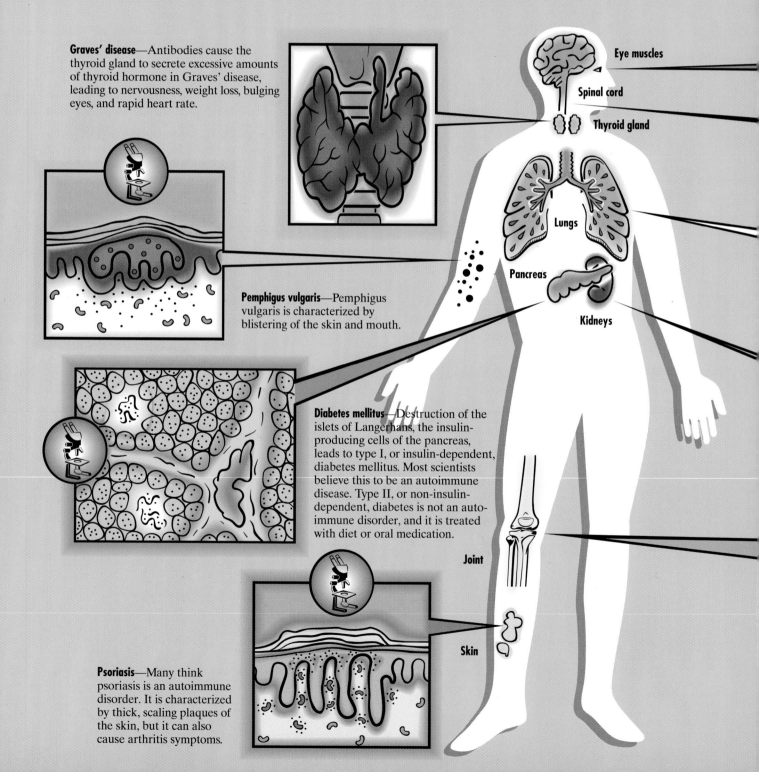

Graves' disease—Antibodies cause the thyroid gland to secrete excessive amounts of thyroid hormone in Graves' disease, leading to nervousness, weight loss, bulging eyes, and rapid heart rate.

Pemphigus vulgaris—Pemphigus vulgaris is characterized by blistering of the skin and mouth.

Diabetes mellitus—Destruction of the islets of Langerhans, the insulin-producing cells of the pancreas, leads to type I, or insulin-dependent, diabetes mellitus. Most scientists believe this to be an autoimmune disease. Type II, or non-insulin-dependent, diabetes is not an auto-immune disorder, and it is treated with diet or oral medication.

Psoriasis—Many think psoriasis is an autoimmune disorder. It is characterized by thick, scaling plaques of the skin, but it can also cause arthritis symptoms.

Eye muscles

Spinal cord

Thyroid gland

Lungs

Pancreas

Kidneys

Joint

Skin

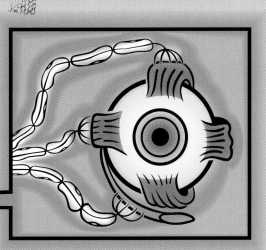

Myasthenia gravis—In myasthenis gravis, immune system cells attack the neuro-muscular junction, which is the site where nerve endings attach to muscle. Weakness of eye and facial musculature is especially common, but limb weakness occurs also.

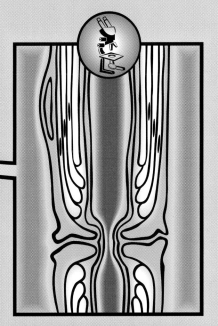

Sarcoidosis—The cause of sarcoidosis is unknown. In this disorder, localized collections of inflammatory cells, called granulomas, accumulate in the lungs, liver, eyes, and skin.

Multiple sclerosis—In multiple sclerosis, immune system cells attack the myelin sheath, the white protective covering of the central nervous system. Symptoms include tingling, muscle weakness, visual disturbances, and loss of coordination.

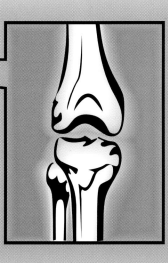

Systemic lupus erythematosus—Systemic lupus erythematosus, or lupus, affects connective tissue in many organs, including muscles, bone, skin, blood, nervous system, heart, lungs, eyes, and kidneys.

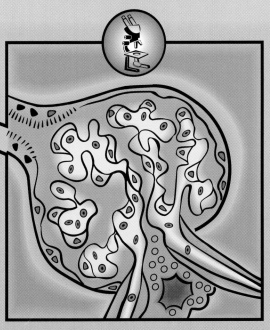

Rheumatoid arthritis—In rheumatoid arthritis, immune system cells attack joint linings, leading to pain and disability.

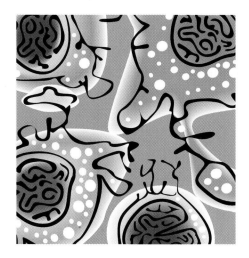

Immune System Cancers I:
The Leukemias

A *NEOPLASM* IS a new and abnormal formation of tissue, such as a tumor or other growth. The word literally means "new form." Some neoplasms are *benign*, meaning that they do not invade other organs or metastasize (spread) to distant body sites, and other neoplasms are *malignant*, meaning that they can metastasize, or spread, to other organs. When referring specifically to malignant neoplasms, people generally use the familiar term *cancer*. Cancer is an uncontrolled proliferation of abnormal cells that flourishes at the expense of the body it inhabits. It can affect any organ system in the body, including the immune system, as we will see in this chapter and the next.

Leukemia is a malignant transformation of the blood-forming cells in the bone marrow and lymphoid organs that, left untreated, eventually replaces normal cells. There are several different types of leukemia, but they share certain characteristics. They all result from the malignant transformation of a single immature blood cell precursor (or "parent" cell) that rapidly divides into identical clones. The clones never advance past the immature stage of development and are released into the circulation, where they can spread to the lymph nodes, spleen, skin, abdominal organs, or central nervous system. The initial malignant transformation can occasionally be linked to a genetic or environmental factor, such as a virus or radiation, but the cause is usually unknown.

There are basically four types of leukemia: *acute lymphocytic leukemia (ALL), acute myelocytic* (also called *myelogenous*) *leukemia (AML), chronic lymphocytic leukemia (CLL),* and *chronic myelocytic* (*myelogenous*) *leukemia (CML)*. Two other types of leukemia, *hairy-cell* and *T-cell leukemia*, are actually variants of CLL. Cells of the chronic leukemias tend to be more mature than those of the acute leukemias, and life expectancy is usually longer in chronic than in acute leukemias. The myelocytic leukemias involve granulocyte precursors, whereas the lymphocytic leukemias involve lymphocyte (T- or B-cell) precursors.

ALL primarily affects young children, whereas AML occurs at all ages. ALL cases involving B-cells outnumber those involving T-cells 3-to-1, with approximately 15% resembling neither cell type. AML has seven subtypes, labeled M1 through M7, depending on the resemblance of the cells to granulocytes, monocytes, erythrocytes, or megakaryocytes. ALL subtypes are classified as L1,

L2, or L3, depending on the uniformity of the cells. AML can be distinguished from ALL by the presence of abnormal granules, called *Auer rods*, that can be seen in the leukemia cells when viewed through a microscope. ALL can be identified by testing for a specific enzyme, called *TdT*, in the laboratory. A particular antigen, called *CALLA*, is also present in 60% of ALL cases and can aid in the diagnosis of this disease.

As a result of the replacement of normal blood cells by malignant cells, people with AML and ALL usually are anemic, have impaired blood clotting abilities, and are especially vulnerable to infections. Pallor, fatigability, easy bruising, spleen and liver enlargement, and bone pain are all common features of these diseases. The abnormal cells can infiltrate other organs, including the kidneys, gastrointestinal tract, and central nervous system. Invasion of the last can lead to *leukemic meningitis*, a condition characterized by headaches, nausea and vomiting, seizures, and decreased ability to think clearly.

Treatment for ALL and AML usually takes place in three stages. First, an abatement of symptoms, *remission,* is attempted by administering potent drugs (chemotherapy) to reduce the number of malignant cells to an undetectable level. Once remission is achieved, more chemotherapy is given to further reduce the number of leukemia cells; this is the *consolidation* phase. Finally, *maintenance* chemotherapy is given for several years to prevent a relapse. Occasionally, radiation therapy is directed at sites where abnormal cells congregate in unusually high numbers. Transfusions of red blood cells and platelets are given as needed to correct anemia and clotting dysfunction. Aggressive treatment of infections and observance of aseptic (sterile) technique on the part of health care personnel, such as wearing masks and gloves and hand-washing, are also essential. Bone marrow transplantation is a treatment option for some people with AML or ALL, especially when an identical twin donor is available. This procedure will be discussed in greater detail in Chapter 17.

Survival in AML and ALL depends on several factors. An initial remission can be achieved in most cases, but with each relapse, the chances of obtaining another remission diminish significantly. Children generally fare better than adults. Approximately 50% of children can expect to live five or more years after diagnosis, whereas less than 20% of adults will do the same.

The chronic leukemias are seen almost exclusively in adults, with 45 to 60 years being the average age. CLL is characterized by an accumulation of mature-appearing B-cells that infiltrate the bone marrow, spleen, and lymph nodes. Symptoms include anemia, lymph node enlargement, and susceptibility to infection. Some people with

CLL can also develop an immunohemolytic anemia, which was discussed in Chapter 12. Survival can exceed 10 years in cases of CLL that affect fewer than three lymph node groups, regardless of treatment interventions. Involvement of more than three lymph node groups or a severe depression of blood and platelet counts generally signifies a worse prognosis, so chemotherapy is usually implemented in these cases to control symptoms and reduce the number of abnormal cells; remission, however, is seldom achieved.

A rare form of CLL involves T-cells rather than B-cells. It is called *T-cell leukemia* and is caused by a virus that is closely related to the AIDS virus. T-cell leukemia is characterized by skin infiltration, enlarged lymph nodes, and an elevated level of calcium in the blood. Attempts to treat this disease usually have little effect.

Hairy-cell leukemia is a B-cell leukemia that is named for the characteristic "spikes" seen on the individual cells. Enlargement of the spleen is common in this disease, as are blood vessel inflammation, blood count depression, and susceptibility to infection. In fact, opportunistic infections, meaning those which take advantage of a person's weakened immune system, are the primary cause of death in people with hairy-cell leukemia. Removal of the spleen is the most effective treatment for this illness. Those who fail to respond to this intervention may benefit from treatment with *alpha interferon*. This protein is similar to the *beta interferon* mentioned in Chapter 14. Some experimental drugs also show promise as possible treatments for hairy-cell leukemia.

The other chronic leukemia, CML, usually progresses in two phases. During the *chronic phase*, there is a marked increase in the number of granulocytes, especially neutrophils, along with anemia, weight loss, fever, and enlargement of the spleen. The chronic phase can be interrupted by an *acute phase*, or *blast crisis*, which resembles AML. During a blast crisis, there is a rapid proliferation of immature granulocyte precursor cells. There is no way to predict when a blast crisis will occur, and it is usually during this phase that people succumb to the illness.

CML can be easily diagnosed, not only on the basis of the enlarged spleen and elevated white blood cell count, but also by the presence of a specific genetic abnormality, called the *Philadelphia chromosome*. People with CML can survive for long periods of time if blast crises can be avoided through the use of chemotherapy. Bone marrow transplantation is also effective if performed in the absence of a blast crisis. Researchers are currently investigating agents that attack CML at the genetic level, as well as alpha interferon, which may have a role in treating this disease

Leukemia

Leukemia is a malignant transformation and uncontrolled multiplication of immature blood cell precursors that thrive at the expense of normal cells. All abnormal cells in leukemia are identical clones of the original malignant cell. As the disease progresses, it impairs the body's ability to make normal blood cells and fight off infection. Leukemia, especially when acute, often proves fatal as it spreads to other organs.

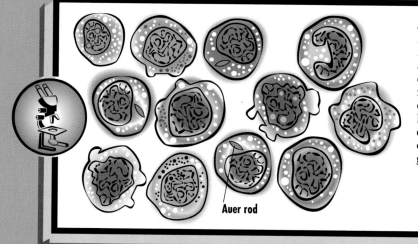

Auer rod

Acute myelocytic leukemia (AML)
Acute myelocytic leukemia, or AML, affects people of all ages and is classified into seven subtypes, depending on whether the cells resemble granulocytes, monocytes, erythrocytes, or megakaryocytes. Many, but not all, cases of AML can be identified by the presence of Auer rods, which are abnormal granules within the leukemic cells.

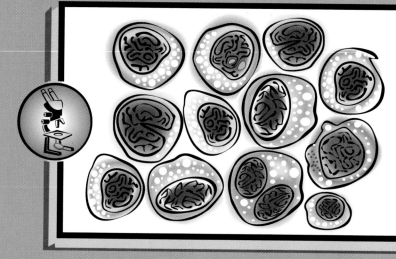

Acute lymphocytic leukemia (ALL)
Acute lymphocytic leukemia, or ALL, occurs primarily in children. Most of the abnormal cells are of the B-cell type, though some are of the T-cell variety. As with AML, the leukemic cells of ALL replace normal blood cells, causing anemia, clotting dysfunction, and susceptibility to opportunistic infections.

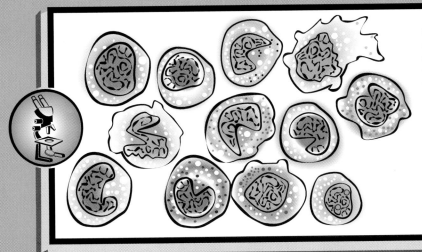

Chronic myelocytic leukemia (CML)

Chronic myelocytic leukemia, or CML, can be detected with relative ease because of a characteristic genetic abnormality called the Philadelphia chromosome. During a blast crisis, an acute episode that resembles AML, people with CML become much sicker and may die. If treatment is successful in controlling blast crises, people with CML can live a long time.

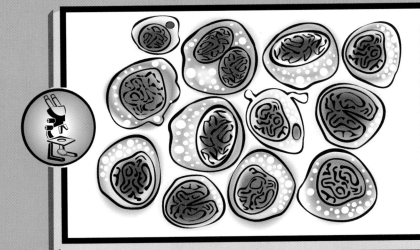

Chronic lymphocytic leukemia (CLL)

Chronic lymphocytic leukemia, or CLL, is the mildest of the leukemias. In fact, treatment is not even necessary in instances where blood counts are relatively normal and only a few lymph node groups are affected. Abnormal B-cells predominate in most cases of CLL, but there is a rare form of CLL called T-cell leukemia.

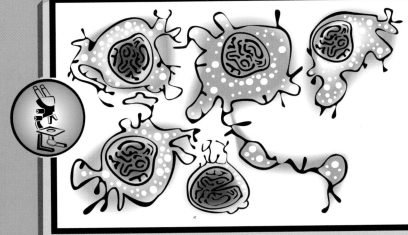

Hairy-cell leukemia

Hairy-cell leukemia is a subtype of CLL and is named for the hair-like projections seen on the abnormal B-cells in this disease.

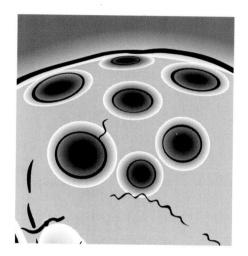

CHAPTER 16

Immune System Cancers II: The Lymphomas and Multiple Myeloma

LYMPHOMA IS A general term used to describe any neoplasm arising in the lymphatic or reticuloendothelial system (RES). Traditionally, lymphomas have been classified as *Hodgkin's* or *non-Hodgkin's* types, with the latter group also referred to as *lymphosarcoma*, or *malignant lymphoma*. More sophisticated diagnostic techniques have led to the more accurate classifications of Hodgkin's and *lymphocytic* lymphomas. Two rare forms of lymphoma, *Burkitt's lymphoma* and *mycosis fungoides*, are included in the lymphocytic lymphoma group.

Lymphomas arise in the lymph nodes and in the lymphoid portions of the gastrointestinal tract, lungs, and skin. Most (90%) Hodgkin's lymphomas begin in the lymph nodes, whereas only 60% of lymphocytic lymphomas arise here. The cause of Hodgkin's disease is unknown, but several lymphocytic lymphomas can originate with a viral infection. There also appears to be a tendency for these illnesses to run in families, though usually they are not directly heritable.

The first signs of Hodgkin's disease can be either a painless enlargement of the lymph nodes or fever, night sweats, and weight loss. Those people whose disease begins without symptoms usually fare better than those who have these complaints from the outset. As the disease progresses, cells spread to neighboring lymph node groups and begin to invade other structures, including the lungs, blood vessels, liver, and abdominal organs. Bone marrow involvement is frequently seen and can lead to pain, displacement of normal cells, anemia, buildup of extra bone, and compression of the spinal cord, which can result in paraplegia. People with Hodgkin's disease also typically have defects in cell-mediated (T-cell) immune function, though antibody production is usually normal. As a result of these defects, a greater tendency toward infection, especially by opportunistic organisms, exists.

In order for a doctor to diagnose Hodgkin's disease, a biopsy specimen of the tumor must be taken and examined under the microscope to see whether the characteristic *Reed-Sternberg cell* is present. If it is, additional tests, such as x-rays, CAT scans, and blood tests, are performed to determine the extent of the disease. If only one or two lymph node groups are affected, radiation therapy can cure the disease. More advanced Hodgkin's lymphomas may require chemotherapy or bone marrow transplantation, but chances of survival are still good. Research into directing natural killer (NK) cells specifically against Hodgkin's lymphoma cells is currently taking place.

Of the lymphocytic lymphomas, 65% are of the B-cell type and 35% are of the T-cell type. In fact, you may have already noticed that most of the lymphocytic immune system cancers involve B- rather than T-cells. This is because most T-cells are produced early in life, whereas B-cells are generated throughout life.

Like Hodgkin's lymphoma, the lymphocytic lymphomas can begin as painless lymph node enlargements, but 40% arise instead in body organs. However, widespread dissemination of the malignant cells is seen earlier and more frequently than it is in Hodgkin's disease. As a result, the severity of disease is determined by the architecture of the cells themselves rather than by the extent of tumor spread. Additionally, immune system function appears to be less affected in the lymphocytic lymphomas than it is in Hodgkin's lymphoma.

The cell types in the lymphocytic lymphomas are classified as low, intermediate, or high grade, with the last carrying the worst prognosis. As with Hodgkin's disease, the diagnosis is made by examining a biopsy sample under the microscope. For the more favorable cell types, radiation with or without chemotherapy can cure about half of lymphocytic lymphomas. More advanced disease is associated with a lower success rate, but bone marrow transplantation may be helpful in these instances.

Burkitt's lymphoma is a rare lymphocytic lymphoma that occurs mostly in people who live in Africa. It is a B-cell tumor that can follow infection with the *Epstein-Barr virus*, the same virus responsible for *mononucleosis*. The cancer arises in the jawbone and can grow to become very large and painful. It is very responsive to chemotherapy if detected early.

Another rare lymphocytic lymphoma, *mycosis fungoides*, is a T-cell tumor that begins in the skin and can spread to other areas. It typically affects people who are over 50 years of age. Chances of survival are excellent, thanks to radiation and topical chemotherapeutic medication. A form of mycosis fungoides, called *Sézary's syndrome*, resembles leukemia. It is characterized by the proliferation of abnormal cells with twisted nuclei in the blood and skin. People with Sézary's syndrome usually have red, itchy, flaking skin and enlarged lymph nodes. As is true of mycosis fungoides, the T-cells in Sézary's syndrome are usually of the helper subtype.

Quite different from the lymphomas is *multiple myeloma*, an uncontrolled proliferation of plasma cell clones that produce a single antibody type and eat away at bone, especially in the pelvis, spine, ribs, and skull. The erosion of bone is accomplished by the activation of bone-eating cells, called *osteoclasts*, which release calcium from the bone into the circulation, causing a marked elevation in the blood calcium level, which is a distinctive feature of this disease. Excessive calcium, in turn, leads to kidney failure, which is compounded by the excretion of antibody pieces called *Bence Jones proteins*.

In addition to bone pain and kidney disease, people with multiple myeloma also tend to be anemic, with clotting abnormalities and blood that is too thick to flow freely through tiny blood vessels. Despite the fact that the myeloma cells secrete antibody, there is a significantly decreased production and increased destruction of normal antibody, leading to an overall lessening in immune system protection. As a result, people with multiple myeloma tend to be especially vulnerable to bacterial infections.

The breakdown of normal antibody in multiple myeloma leads to a rise in the level of antibody pieces called *M component*. Therefore, the presence of M component in the blood or urine is one of the criteria used in the diagnosis of this disease. Plasma cell proliferation in the bone marrow, erosion of bone, and excretion of urinary Bence Jones proteins are also used for this purpose. The severity of the disease depends on the level of calcium and M component in the blood, the degree of anemia, and the extent of bone destruction seen in x-rays. Survival ranges from one to two years in people with stage III myeloma, to five years or more in those with stage I disease. Treatment involves the use of chemotherapeutic drugs, but it is also important to specifically address the elevated calcium level and any kidney damage that might be present, since these factors affect the outcome as well. Alpha interferon is increasingly gaining favor as an additional modality in treating multiple myeloma.

Lymphoma and Multiple Myeloma

Lymphomas are malignancies of the lymphatic and reticuloendothelial (RES) systems. They arise in the lymph nodes or in the lymphoid tissues of the lungs, skin, and gastro-intestinal tract. As with any type of cancer, lymphomas can spread to other organs if left untreated.

Multiple myeloma
Multiple myeloma is a malignant proliferation of plasma cells that produce abnormal antibody at the expense of normal antibody. People with this disease tend to have kidney failure, bone pain, and depressed immune system function.

Activation of osteoclasts, which are cells that eat bone, is characteristic of multiple myeloma. The areas of bone destruction can be seen as "punched-out" areas on an x-ray.

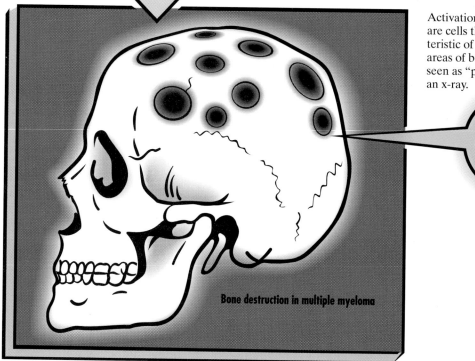

Osteoclast

Bone destruction in multiple myeloma

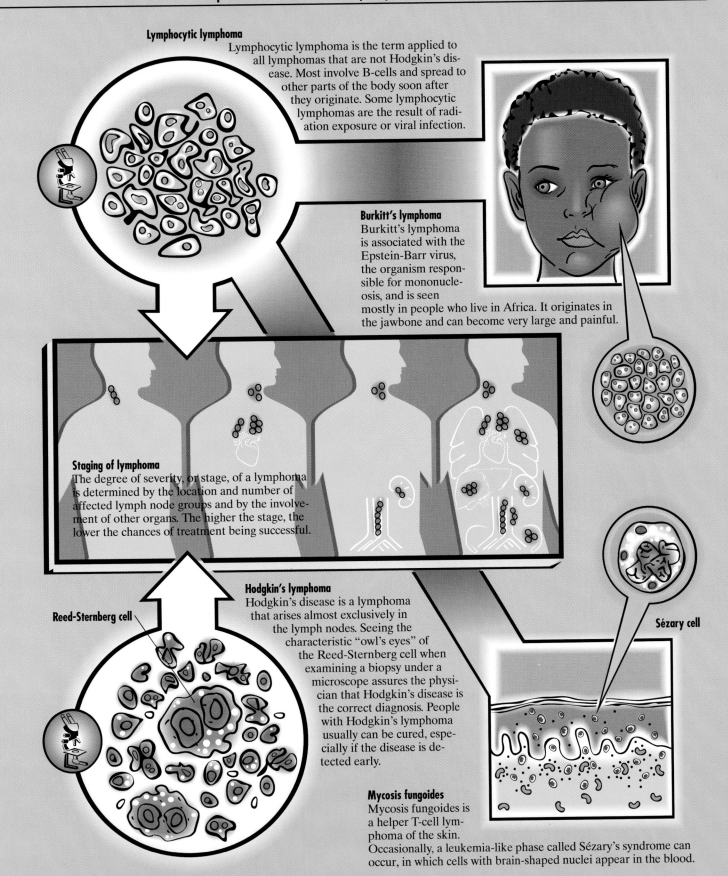

Lymphocytic lymphoma

Lymphocytic lymphoma is the term applied to all lymphomas that are not Hodgkin's disease. Most involve B-cells and spread to other parts of the body soon after they originate. Some lymphocytic lymphomas are the result of radiation exposure or viral infection.

Burkitt's lymphoma

Burkitt's lymphoma is associated with the Epstein-Barr virus, the organism responsible for mononucleosis, and is seen mostly in people who live in Africa. It originates in the jawbone and can become very large and painful.

Staging of lymphoma

The degree of severity, or stage, of a lymphoma is determined by the location and number of affected lymph node groups and by the involvement of other organs. The higher the stage, the lower the chances of treatment being successful.

Reed-Sternberg cell

Hodgkin's lymphoma

Hodgkin's disease is a lymphoma that arises almost exclusively in the lymph nodes. Seeing the characteristic "owl's eyes" of the Reed-Sternberg cell when examining a biopsy under a microscope assures the physician that Hodgkin's disease is the correct diagnosis. People with Hodgkin's lymphoma usually can be cured, especially if the disease is detected early.

Sézary cell

Mycosis fungoides

Mycosis fungoides is a helper T-cell lymphoma of the skin. Occasionally, a leukemia-like phase called Sézary's syndrome can occur, in which cells with brain-shaped nuclei appear in the blood.

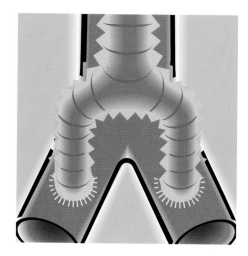

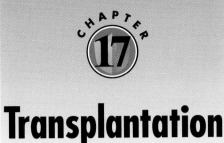

Transplantation

BODY ORGANS ARE affected by an immense variety of disease processes. Some of these diseases are so severe that they literally destroy their target organ. When this occurs, it is often necessary to replace the damaged organ with a healthy one in order to save the life of the individual or prevent a permanent disability. This swapping of organs is called *transplantation*.

The organ or tissue that is transplanted is called a *graft*. There are five types of grafts. First, the form of transplantation with which most people are familiar is the *allograft*, or *homograft*. This is a transplant that occurs between two individuals of the same species. Removal of the heart from a donor who has suffered brain death and the subsequent insertion of the heart into the body of a recipient is an example of an allograft. Other organs that have been allografted include the pancreas, bone marrow, cornea, small intestine, liver, and lung. A single kidney that is removed from a living donor for transplantation purposes is also an allograft. However, a kidney harvested from an identical twin donor is not an allograft but an *isograft*, or *syngeneic graft*, because its HLA antigens are identical to those of the recipient and are recognized as "self" by the recipient's immune system.

The third type of graft is the *autograft*, or *autogenous graft*, which is taken from one area of a person's body and moved to another area on the same body. Skin grafts for the treatment of burn victims, tendon and bone grafts for orthopedic procedures, flaps of muscle and skin for plastic surgery reconstructions, and vein grafts for coronary artery bypass surgery are all examples of autografts.

Organs for transplantation can be taken not only from other people but also from other species of animals. This fourth graft type is the *xenograft*, or *heterograft*. Heart valves from pigs are xenografts that are routinely used to replace faulty human heart valves. Foreign antigens are removed from such grafts before they are inserted. Temporary xenografts, such as baboon liver transplants, have been used on rare occasions. The final type of graft is the *synthetic graft*, in which artificial materials are inserted to augment or replace the function of a native structure.

Allografts and xenografts are regarded as foreign by the recipient's immune system and are attacked. This process is called *rejection*, and as we learned in Chapter 13, it is the result of the immune system's detection of unfamiliar HLA antigens. Most instances of rejection are caused by

T-cells that become sensitized to the foreign antigen in a manner resembling the type IV hypersensitivity reactions discussed in Chapter 12. This is called *acute rejection*. Sometimes a transplant recipient is presensitized to antigens contained in the graft and rejects the organ in a matter of minutes or hours. This is *hyperacute rejection* and is a form of type II hypersensitivity, another concept covered in Chapter 12.

Although there is no way to halt the progression of hyperacute rejection, drugs are available to minimize the effects of acute rejection. However, even when these medications are successful in staving off immune system defenses, after several years, a certain degree of *chronic rejection* is inevitable. In this process, the accumulation of scar tissue gradually encroaches upon the organ's blood supply.

To ensure the best possible outcome in an organ transplantation, the HLA antigens of the donor and of the recipient must be matched as closely as possible. Techniques such as leukocyte typing, cross-matching, and mixed lymphocyte culturing all involve the combining of various quantities of serum and cells from the donor and from the recipient in order to determine HLA compatibility. Only in the case of isografting, in which the donor and recipient are identical twins, can perfect tissue compatibility occur. A close relative may possess the same set of HLA antigens as the prospective recipient, but rejection of the transplanted organ will still take place. This is because other antigens besides those of the HLA type play a role in determining tissue compatibility. However, the optimal degree of transplant success is usually obtained when organs are harvested from a close relative, even if the HLA match is inferior to that of a stranger's organ.

Once transplantion has taken place, *immunosuppression therapy* must be initiated in the attempt to prevent rejection of the graft by the recipient's immune system. A variety of drugs are used to inhibit the proliferation of T- and B-cells that are targeted against the transplanted organ. These include antimetabolites, alkylating agents, immunosuppresive antibiotics, and cyclosporine. These same drugs are also used in various cancer chemotherapy regimens. In addition to drugs that block the proliferation of T- and B-cells, adrenocorticosteroids, such as prednisone, are usually part of an anti-rejection treatment regimen. Steroids not only decrease the number of T- and B-cells, but they also suppress inflammation and inhibit the activity of phagocytes.

Immunosuppression therapy is indiscriminate; it affects the entire immune system, not just the cells that target a transplanted organ. As a result, people taking these types of medication are vulnerable to opportunistic infections and to certain malignancies, such as lymphoma, cervical cancer, and skin cancer. In addition, people taking steroids for extended periods of time usually develop *Cushing's syndrome*, a phenomenon that is characterized by roundness of the face, obesity of the torso, "buffalo hump" formation at the base of the neck, thinness and fragility of the skin, and impaired wound-healing ability. Other consequences of immunosuppression therapy include gastrointestinal bleeding, cataracts, thrombophlebitis, hypertension, metabolic imbalances, pancreatitis, and kidney damage.

Bone marrow transplantation deserves special consideration because it is unlike any other type of transplant. Used in the treatment of genetic blood disorders, immune system malignancies, and *aplastic anemia*, the transplant procedure itself is quite simple. Toxic chemotherapeutic drugs are administered, often in conjunction with radiation, with the intent of destroying the recipient's defective bone marrow. Healthy bone marrow is then removed from the donor's body and infused into the recipient's. Ideally, the transplanted bone marrow produces normal blood cells and the recipient is cured of the disease. Thus, bone marrow transplantation is unique because it is the only form of transplantation that produces a *chimera*, which is an individual whose body contains living, proliferating cells of a different genetic origin.

Not only is the transplantation of bone marrow distinctive, so is the rejection of bone marrow grafts. Unlike other allografts, where the recipient's immune system will reject the transplanted organ, bone marrow transplantation essentially gives the recipient a new immune system. Therefore, when rejection occurs, it is the graft that targets the body receiving it, rather than vice versa. This is called *graft-versus-host disease (GVHD)* and is the most significant problem encountered in bone marrow transplantation.

GVHD is manifested in the form of skin rashes, diarrhea, abdominal pain, liver involvement, and susceptibility to opportunistic infection. Some cases of GVHD are mild, but up to one-third of the more severe incidences are fatal. GVHD is not a factor in a bone marrow *autograft*, which is a technique that is undertaken following radiation and chemotherapy for leukemia and lymphoma as a means of reversing the bone marrow depletion that results. In this procedure, an unaffected portion of a person's own marrow is removed and frozen. Once therapy has been completed, the bone marrow is thawed and reinfused. Current research is focusing on the creation of antibodies that counteract the T-cells responsible for GVHD.

Graft Types

Allograft

An organ that is transplanted from one person to another is called an allograft. Many different organs have been transplanted with varying degrees of success, including the heart, kidney, cornea, bone marrow, pancreas, liver, lung, and small intestine. Allograft donors are classified as either living or cadaver donors.

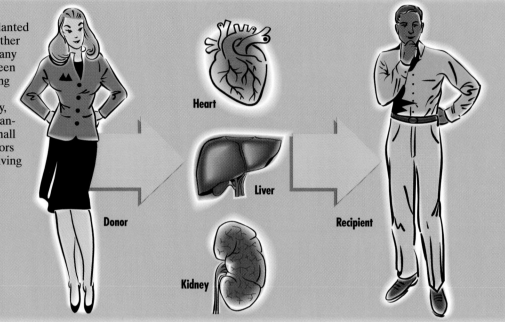

Heart

Liver

Kidney

Donor

Recipient

Isograft

An isograft is the same as an allograft, except that the donor and recipient are identical twins. Identical twins share the same genetic code and, consequently, the same HLA antigens. For this reason, isografts are recognized as "self" by the recipient's immune system and are not rejected.

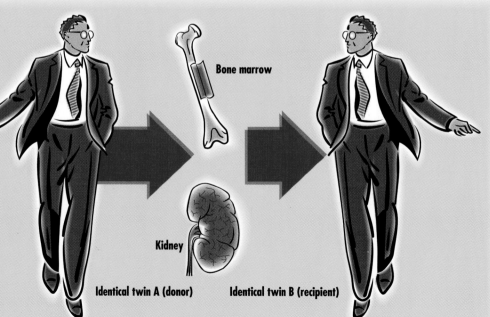

Bone marrow

Kidney

Identical twin A (donor)   Identical twin B (recipient)

Autograft

Autografts are not rejected, because they are composed of tissue that is moved from one part of the body to another part of the same body.

Flaps of muscle and skin, called myocutaneous flaps, are used in situations ranging from breast reconstruction to coverage of bedsores.

Myocutaneous flap

Skin graft

Vein graft

Many coronary artery bypass operations utilize a segment of the saphenous vein in the leg to form a detour around the occluded heart vessel.

Skin grafts are frequently used to cover severe burns or other wounds. A thin piece of skin is removed from the donor site, usually the thigh, back, or buttock, and attached to the injured area.

Synthetic Graft

Synthetic materials are increasingly being used to assist or replace organs or structures that have ceased to function properly.

Xenograft

A xenogaft is an organ or tissue that is removed from an animal and transplanted into a human.

Valve from pig

Porcine (pig) heart valves, used to replace faulty human heart valves, are composed of nonliving tissue and can therefore be cleansed of all foreign HLA antigens.

Xenografts of living tissue, such as a baboon liver, are temporary and are utilized solely as a means of "buying time" until a compatible human donor organ can be found.

Liver from baboon

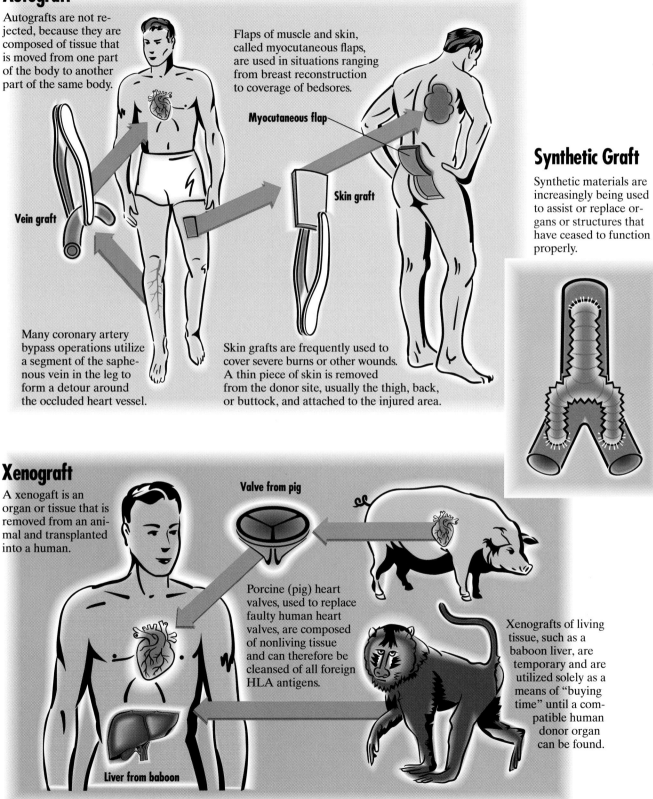

Graft Rejection

Acute Rejection

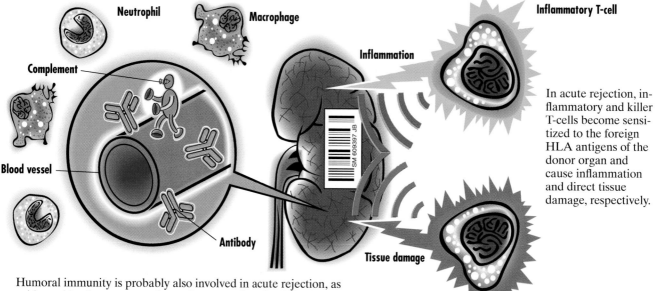

Neutrophil

Macrophage

Complement

Inflammation

Inflammatory T-cell

Blood vessel

Antibody

SM 609397 JB

Tissue damage

Killer T-cell

In acute rejection, inflammatory and killer T-cells become sensitized to the foreign HLA antigens of the donor organ and cause inflammation and direct tissue damage, respectively.

Humoral immunity is probably also involved in acute rejection, as evidenced by the presence of complement and antibody in the blood vessels of the donor organ. Macrophages and neutrophils infiltrate the foreign tissue, but the blood vessels remain open.

Chronic Rejection

Scar tissue

Blood vessel

Hyperacute rejection is rare, thanks to advances in tissue cross-matching, and acute rejection can usually be controlled through the use of immunosuppression therapy. However, a certain degree of chronic rejection inevitably follows transplantation. Characteristic of this type of reaction is scar tissue that gradually chokes off the donor organ's blood supply. Eosinophils and plasma cells are abundant in the surrounding the area.

Plasma cell

Eosinophil

Bone Marrow Transplantation

The first step in bone marrow transplantation is ablation, which is destruction of the recipient's diseased marrow with toxic chemotherapeutic drugs and radiation.

Chemotherapy

Radiation

Following ablation of the recipient's bone marrow, healthy marrow is collected from the donor's body and infused into the recipient's.

Recipient

Donor

Hyperacute Rejection

A previous transplant, pregnancy, or transfusion can cause the formation of antibodies to HLA antigens contained in the donor organ. When transplantation is attempted, the antibodies rapidly attach to the organ and signal neutrophils to destroy it.

Preformed antibodies

Neutrophil

Microscopically, hyperacute rejection resembles a type II hypersensitivity reaction, with complement and antigen-antibody complexes in the walls of the blood vessels. In a matter of hours, or even minutes, blood clots form within the donor organ's blood vessels, thus cutting off its blood supply.

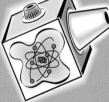

Complement

Blood clot

Antibody

Blood vessel

Graft-vs.-Host Disease (GVHD)

Opportunistic infection

Graft-versus-host disease is the most significant complication of bone marrow transplantation. Healthy T-cells that arise from the donated marrow identify the recipient's body as foreign tissue and launch an attack against it. Symptoms include diarrhea, abdominal pain, liver dysfunction, skin rash, and opportunistic infections. Severe cases of graft-versus-host disease are often fatal.

Liver

Skin

Intestines

T-cell

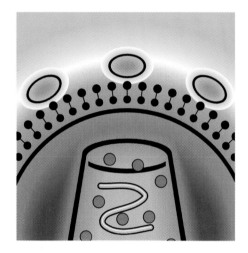

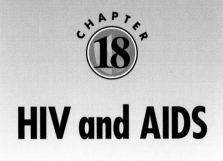

HIV and AIDS

THE *HUMAN IMMUNODEFICIENCY VIRUS (HIV)*, the virus that causes AIDS, probably is the most intensively studied virus in history. The reason this particular infectious organism has attracted so much attention from both the public and the health care communities is due to the numerous social implications that accompany an infection with HIV. Discovered in the early 1980s, the virus has greatly affected not only the practice of health care, but interpersonal relationships as well. Estimates of the number of people in the United States who are infected with HIV vary from source to source, but it is undoubtedly more than one million.

HIV belongs to the *retrovirus* family of RNA viruses, a group that is unique in its ability to create DNA using RNA. HIV primarily infects T-cells, especially those of the helper and inflammatory subtypes, but it can also invade monocytes, macrophages, and other types of cells. A healthy immune system can keep an HIV invasion under control for years; killer T-cells destroy infected cells, and B-cells create antibodies against the virus. However, the progressive loss of helper T-cells not only leads to a deficiency in immune system protection, but it also results in a relative surplus of suppressor T-cells, which further depress the body's defensive capabilities.

Once a person becomes infected with HIV, it takes two or more months for the immune system to form antibodies to the organism. When these antibodies reach a blood level that can be detected by laboratory tests, the person is said to have *seroconverted* and a diagnosis of HIV infection can be made with certainty. Following seroconversion, an infected person is said to be HIV-positive. During the months that elapse between infection with HIV and seroconversion, the infected person unknowingly carries the virus and can transmit it to another person. If HIV testing is not performed, a person could carry the virus for years before the development of symptoms.

The stage of HIV infection during which the first symptoms appear is called the *AIDS-related complex (ARC)*. It initially resembles a flu-like illness with symptoms that include fever, enlarged lymph nodes, fatigue, weakness, and weight loss. As the immune system sustains further damage, more severe weight loss, diarrhea, and oral fungal infections occur. The emergence of opportunistic infections (those which take advantage of a person's weakened immune system) signifies the onset of the *acquired immunodeficiency syndrome*, or *full-blown AIDS*.

Several specific organisms are responsible for the majority of opportunistic infections in people with AIDS. *Pneumocystis carinii* is a microscopic parasite that is present in the lungs of most people, but it is unable to cause problems in those with a normally functioning immune system. However, when the immune system is severely damaged, as in the case of AIDS, the parasite takes advantage of the situation and multiplies, leading to a pneumonia that often is fatal. Another lung infection that is common in people with AIDS is caused by a bacterium called *Mycobacterium avium-intracellulare (MAI)*. MAI infection resembles tuberculosis and is responsible for many AIDS-related deaths. Infections of the central nervous system by opportunistic organisms such as *Toxoplasma gondii*, a parasite, and *Cryptococcus neoformans*, a fungus, are also associated with a high fatality rate and are used as important indicators of the progression of HIV infection from ARC to AIDS. Viruses such as *cytomegalovirus (CMV)* are among the many other organisms that can cause opportunistic infections in people with AIDS.

In addition to opportunistic infections, people with AIDS are susceptible to a specific type of cancer that was rare before the HIV epidemic generated a resurgence. Called *Kaposi's sarcoma*, it is a neoplasm that appears in the form of multiple purple-red nodules that initially erupt on the skin, but later can spread to other organs, including the lungs, lymph nodes, mouth, and gastrointestinal tract. Certain types of lymphoma also are seen frequently in people with AIDS, another consequence of the immune system's inability to mount an effective defense against enemy cells.

Efforts to understand the means by which HIV is transmitted have been clouded by many popular misconceptions. The virus reproduces by invading the interior of T-cells. Therefore, the passing of infected T-cells from one person to another simultaneously transmits the virus. For this to occur, a body fluid that contains T-cells must first exit the body of an infected person. T-cells are found in blood, semen, vaginal secretions, tears, and saliva, although the last two have not been associated with HIV transmission. The infected fluid must then enter the body of an uninfected person. This can be accomplished either through injection, as in the case of needle-sharing among IV drug users, or by contact with a mucous membrane, such as the vagina or the lining of the rectum. The latter route of transmission is especially likely if the mucous membrane is inflamed or injured.

What is important to remember is that HIV is transmitted by an intimate exchange of body fluids. It is not transmitted by casual contact, such as handshaking, nor is it transmitted via inanimate objects, such as toilet seats. The spread of HIV through blood transfusion has become a rarity since routine antibody testing of the blood supply began in the mid-1980s.

The HIV virion itself has features common to all viruses, as well as certain unique characteristics that allow it to reproduce efficiently. The genetic material, in the form of two strands of RNA, is contained within a megaphone-shaped core. Also included within the core is a chemical called *reverse transcriptase*, which is the enzyme that allows the virus's RNA to create DNA once it has invaded a body cell. The core and its contents are protected by an outer double-layered envelope. Protein "studs" cover the surface of the outer envelope and are the means by which the HIV virion attaches to a target cell and injects its genetic material.

Once an HIV particle has attached to a body cell, such as a helper T-cell, it injects its core into the cell's interior, where DNA is created from the viral RNA. This virus-produced DNA then inserts itself into the T-cell's own DNA, resulting in an entirely new genetic code that is capable of manufacturing multiple copies of HIV RNA. The RNA copies move to the surface of the T-cell and, as they push through the cell's outer membrane, wrap themselves in a protective envelope.

The manufacture of viral DNA by reverse transcriptase is the most crucial phase of the reproductive process, because it is this step that has allowed HIV to thwart all attempts medical science has made to combat it. The enzyme makes periodic mistakes when using the virus's RNA to create new DNA, resulting in a completely different genetic code. As a consequence, a new mutation of the original virus is generated—one that is not affected by drugs that may have been effective against its predecessor. Drugs such as AZT and ddI, which have been used in the treatment of AIDS, work by inserting themselves into and arresting the production of virus-manufactured DNA. Over time, however, reverse transcriptase has "learned" to make DNA that ignores the presence of the drug.

Despite more than a decade of exhaustive research and testing of various treatment modalities, a cure or vaccine for HIV continues to elude us. It is the virus's tremendous capacity for mutation that has frustrated our efforts. Current research into creating antibodies that block the attachment of HIV particles to T-cells and into attacking the virus at the genetic level may prove fruitful, but only time will tell. For the present, careful attention to preventive measures, such as avoiding the sharing of syringe needles and abstaining from high-risk sexual practices, is the key to keeping the spread of HIV in check.

HIV Infection

HIV Particle

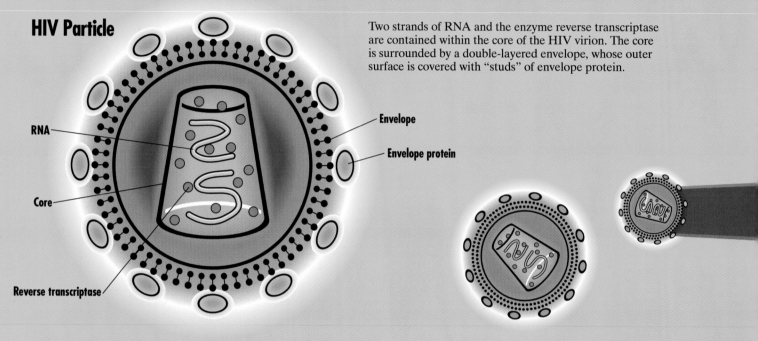

Two strands of RNA and the enzyme reverse transcriptase are contained within the core of the HIV virion. The core is surrounded by a double-layered envelope, whose outer surface is covered with "studs" of envelope protein.

RNA

Core

Reverse transcriptase

Envelope

Envelope protein

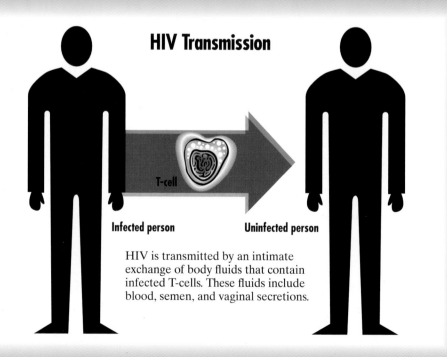

HIV Transmission

T-cell

Infected person

Uninfected person

HIV is transmitted by an intimate exchange of body fluids that contain infected T-cells. These fluids include blood, semen, and vaginal secretions.

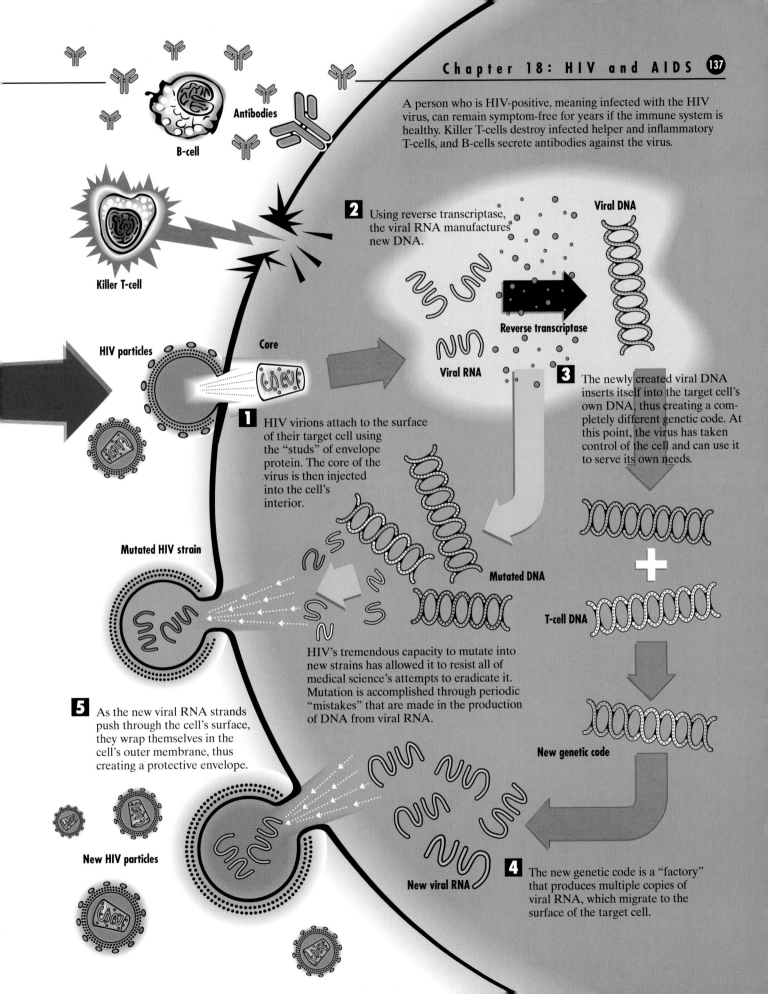

Antibodies

B-cell

Killer T-cell

A person who is HIV-positive, meaning infected with the HIV virus, can remain symptom-free for years if the immune system is healthy. Killer T-cells destroy infected helper and inflammatory T-cells, and B-cells secrete antibodies against the virus.

2 Using reverse transcriptase, the viral RNA manufactures new DNA.

Viral DNA

Reverse transcriptase

Viral RNA

HIV particles

Core

1 HIV virions attach to the surface of their target cell using the "studs" of envelope protein. The core of the virus is then injected into the cell's interior.

3 The newly created viral DNA inserts itself into the target cell's own DNA, thus creating a completely different genetic code. At this point, the virus has taken control of the cell and can use it to serve its own needs.

Mutated HIV strain

Mutated DNA

+

T-cell DNA

HIV's tremendous capacity to mutate into new strains has allowed it to resist all of medical science's attempts to eradicate it. Mutation is accomplished through periodic "mistakes" that are made in the production of DNA from viral RNA.

New genetic code

5 As the new viral RNA strands push through the cell's surface, they wrap themselves in the cell's outer membrane, thus creating a protective envelope.

New HIV particles

New viral RNA

4 The new genetic code is a "factory" that produces multiple copies of viral RNA, which migrate to the surface of the target cell.

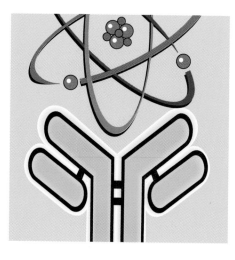

Immunotherapy

MMUNOTHERAPY IS THE utilization of the body's own disease-fighting capabilities to treat illnesses. The field is still in its infancy. Although vaccines for smallpox and rabies were discovered in the 18th and 19th centuries, respectively, most of the vaccines in use today, such as those for polio, mumps, and measles, were developed during the latter part of this century. As important as these discoveries were, even greater discoveries are on the horizon. Scientists have, for a very long time, yearned for the ability to isolate very specific components of the immune system and tailor them to accomplish very specific tasks. Thanks to advances in computer and laboratory technology over the past decade or two, this dream is becoming reality.

Nowhere is the technology explosion more apparent than in the study of *monoclonal antibodies*. In theory, the manufacture of monoclonal antibodies is quite simple. A B-cell that secretes antibody against a desired antigen, such as the vulnerable part of an infectious organism or cancer cell, is isolated and allowed to multiply into numerous identical copies, or clones. The result is a collection of many B-cells, all of which secrete antibody against the same antigen. Ideally, a group of B-cells that secrete antibodies against a certain type of cancer should be able to seek out such a growth within a person's body and destroy it, while leaving the normal body cells alone. As we will discuss in a moment, the actual utilization of monoclonal antibody technology is hampered by several complicating factors.

Monoclonal antibodies can be used by themselves ("naked" antibodies), or they can be linked to other substances and used as "carriers." Used alone, these antibodies attach to their intended target, such as a cancerous growth, and activate complement and the cell-mediated immunity branch into destroying a tumor. In addition, "naked" monoclonal antibodies can be tailor-made to resemble certain antigens, such as cancer cells. They can then be used to stimulate antibody production against the antigen without causing the actual disease associated with the antigen. Attaching a radioactive molecule to a monoclonal antibody and allowing the antibody to find and bind to its target is an excellent way of detecting cancers that are too small to be seen using other methods. Radioactive materials or chemotherapeutic drugs can also be joined to monoclonal antibodies as a means of delivering therapy directly to a tumor.

As with any new technology, the use of monoclonal antibodies has been fraught with problems. The antibodies, on their way from the injection site to their target, must "run the gauntlet" of other body organs, fluids, and tissues. As a result, only a small fraction reaches the intended destination. People treated with monoclonal antibodies typically suffer side effects, such as fever, chills, and serum sickness (see Chapter 12), which result from the formation of antigen-antibody complexes and from the immune system's production of antibodies against the monoclonal antibodies. Chemotherapeutic drugs that are attached to monoclonal antibodies for delivery also have caused their share of problems. It typically takes about two days for a monoclonal antibody to reach its destination. During this interval, the drug maintains contact with normal cells and can exert toxic effects upon them. These problems will undoubtedly be solved, and the future of monoclonal antibody technology remains bright.

A great deal of research is currently devoted to the study of *cytokines* in immunotherapy. This group of naturally occurring hormone-like proteins includes the *interferons* and the *interleukins*. The interferons, which exist in three forms, called alpha, beta, and gamma, are secreted by various cells of the body in response to viral infections. Alpha interferon has attracted a great deal of interest in the area of cancer research. Used experimentally in the treatment of chronic myelogenous leukemia (CML), multiple myeloma, skin cancers such as melanoma, and colon cancer, it has been associated with an impressive success rate. In fact, in the case of CML, alpha interferon actually rids the bone marrow of the *Philadelphia chromosome*, the genetic abnormality responsible for this disease. As we discussed in Chapter 14, beta interferon may be helpful in treating certain autoimmune diseases. The main problem with interferon therapy has been the frequent occurrence of side effects. Ranging from joint pain and weight loss to liver damage and thyroid suppression, these adverse reactions have limited the circumstances under which interferons can be administered.

The interleukins come in many varieties, but it is *interleukin-2 (IL-2)* that has shown the greatest potential as an immunotherapeutic agent. IL-2 is produced by T-cells in response to a foreign invasion and it stimulates the proliferation of B- and T-cells and the production of other cytokines. As with interferons and monoclonal antibodies, its main drawback is the significant number of side effects

Since the early 1980s, scientists have been able to mass-produce IL-2 using genetically engineered bacteria. When cells are taken from the spleen or other lymphoid organs and are incubated with IL-2, a cancer-killing cell called the *lymphokine-activated killer (LAK) cell* is created. When released into the circulation of a person with metastatic cancer (which is cancer that has spread to other sites), LAK cells locate the cancer cells and destroy them, leading to a reduction in the size and number of metastases.

Taking this type of research one step further, scientists are currently investigating *tumor-infiltrating lymphocytes (TIL)*, which are white blood cells that are found within the cancerous growth itself and are highly specific for that cancer type. As a result of this specificity, TILs are many times more effective than LAKs. In the TIL treatment method, the cancer is surgically removed and a small piece is placed beneath the skin near a lymph node. Weeks later, the lymph node is removed and tumor-specific TILs are isolated, cloned, and then injected back into the body, where they attack cancer cells that were missed during surgery.

Immunotherapy research extends far beyond the realm of cancer treatment. One day it may be possible to prevent transplant rejection or autoimmune diseases by presenting specific antigens to immature T-cells in the thymus. Diabetes, and other diseases that are caused by antibodies against "self" tissue, may respond to treatment with *anti-antibodies* that block the problem-causing antibodies and prevent them from exerting their effects. Vaccines for some autoimmune diseases, such as diabetes, multiple sclerosis, and rheumatoid arthritis, may not be far away. These vaccines would work by selectively eliminating the T-cells responsible for a particular disease. Vaccines to combat allergies may be possible as well. Certain interleukins secreted by T-cells are known to exacerbate allergic reactions by stimulating the production of IgE. A vaccine, using gamma-interferon perhaps, may be able to block these interleukins and improve symptoms.

Finally, a great deal of research is being devoted to finding an effective vaccine or treatment regimen for AIDS. Antibodies to the envelope proteins of HIV may yield a vaccine. An even more technologically sophisticated approach involves introducing genetic material that is targeted against the HIV virus into an infected person's T-cells. While no one can know what the future will bring, it is clear that we have seen only the tip of the immunotherapy "iceberg."

Monoclonal Antibodies

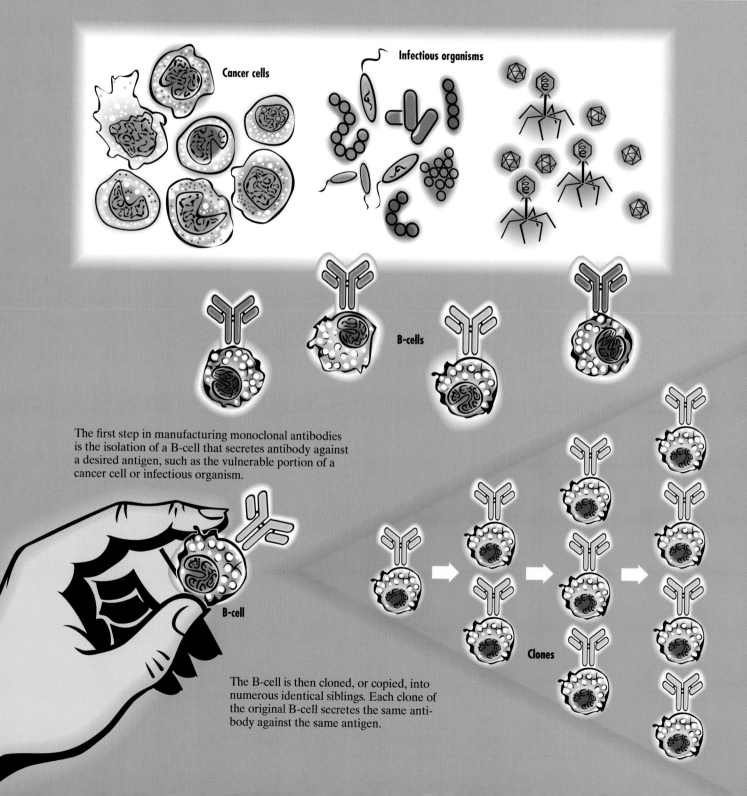

The first step in manufacturing monoclonal antibodies is the isolation of a B-cell that secretes antibody against a desired antigen, such as the vulnerable portion of a cancer cell or infectious organism.

The B-cell is then cloned, or copied, into numerous identical siblings. Each clone of the original B-cell secretes the same antibody against the same antigen.

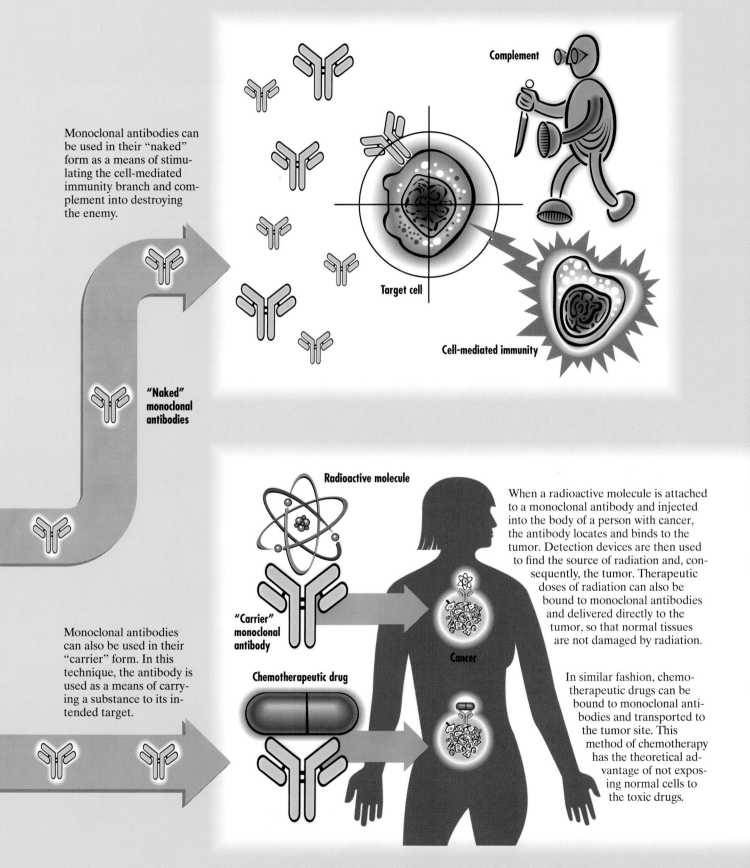

Monoclonal antibodies can be used in their "naked" form as a means of stimulating the cell-mediated immunity branch and complement into destroying the enemy.

Complement

Target cell

Cell-mediated immunity

"Naked" monoclonal antibodies

Monoclonal antibodies can also be used in their "carrier" form. In this technique, the antibody is used as a means of carrying a substance to its intended target.

Radioactive molecule

"Carrier" monoclonal antibody

Chemotherapeutic drug

Cancer

When a radioactive molecule is attached to a monoclonal antibody and injected into the body of a person with cancer, the antibody locates and binds to the tumor. Detection devices are then used to find the source of radiation and, consequently, the tumor. Therapeutic doses of radiation can also be bound to monoclonal antibodies and delivered directly to the tumor, so that normal tissues are not damaged by radiation.

In similar fashion, chemotherapeutic drugs can be bound to monoclonal antibodies and transported to the tumor site. This method of chemotherapy has the theoretical advantage of not exposing normal cells to the toxic drugs.

Cytokines, LAKs, and TILs

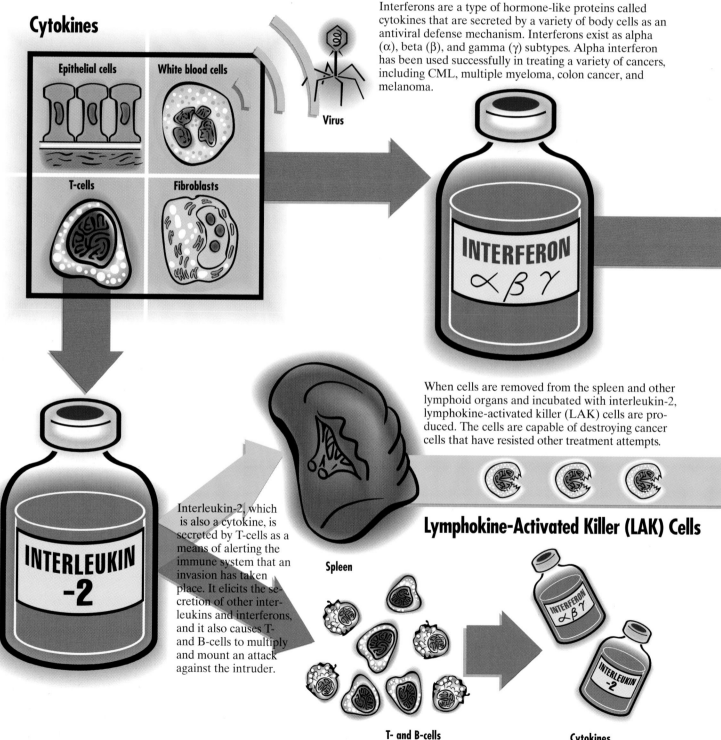

Cytokines

Epithelial cells

White blood cells

T-cells

Fibroblasts

Virus

Interferons are a type of hormone-like proteins called cytokines that are secreted by a variety of body cells as an antiviral defense mechanism. Interferons exist as alpha (α), beta (β), and gamma (γ) subtypes. Alpha interferon has been used successfully in treating a variety of cancers, including CML, multiple myeloma, colon cancer, and melanoma.

INTERFERON αβγ

When cells are removed from the spleen and other lymphoid organs and incubated with interleukin-2, lymphokine-activated killer (LAK) cells are produced. The cells are capable of destroying cancer cells that have resisted other treatment attempts.

INTERLEUKIN-2

Interleukin-2, which is also a cytokine, is secreted by T-cells as a means of alerting the immune system that an invasion has taken place. It elicits the secretion of other interleukins and interferons, and it also causes T- and B-cells to multiply and mount an attack against the intruder.

Spleen

Lymphokine-Activated Killer (LAK) Cells

T- and B-cells

Cytokines

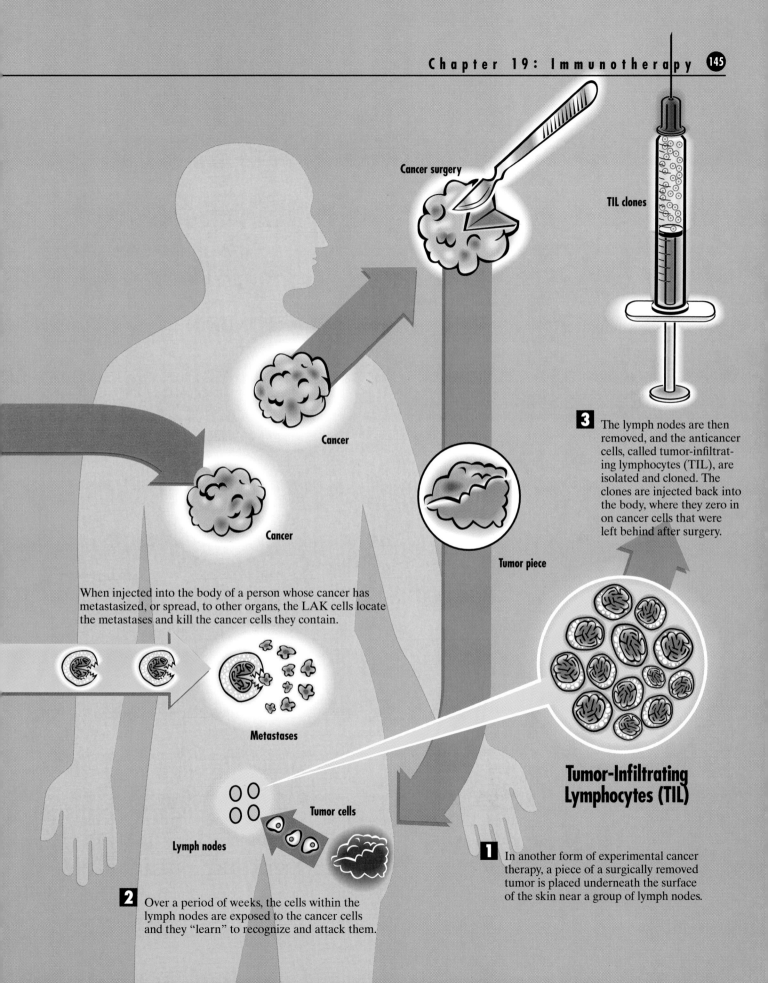

Cancer surgery

TIL clones

Cancer

Cancer

3 The lymph nodes are then removed, and the anticancer cells, called tumor-infiltrating lymphocytes (TIL), are isolated and cloned. The clones are injected back into the body, where they zero in on cancer cells that were left behind after surgery.

Tumor piece

When injected into the body of a person whose cancer has metastasized, or spread, to other organs, the LAK cells locate the metastases and kill the cancer cells they contain.

Metastases

Tumor-Infiltrating Lymphocytes (TIL)

Tumor cells

Lymph nodes

1 In another form of experimental cancer therapy, a piece of a surgically removed tumor is placed underneath the surface of the skin near a group of lymph nodes.

2 Over a period of weeks, the cells within the lymph nodes are exposed to the cancer cells and they "learn" to recognize and attack them.

ATTENTION TEACHERS AND TRAINERS
Now You Can Teach From These Books!

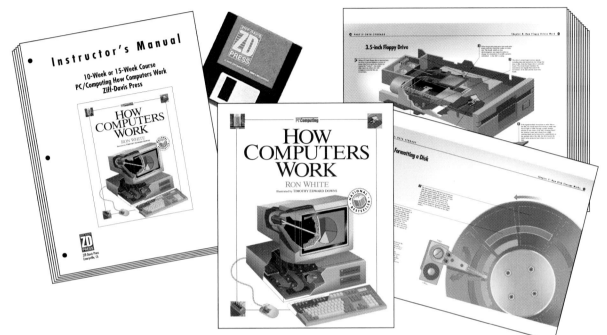

ZD Press now offers instructors and trainers
the materials they need to use these books in their classes.

- An Instructor's Manual features flexible lessons designed for use in a
  10- or 15-week course (30-45 course hours).

- Student exercises and tests on floppy disk provide you with an
  easy way to tailor and/or duplicate tests as you need them.

- A Transparency Package contains all the graphics from the book, each
  on a single, full-color transparency.

- Spanish edition of *PC/Computing How Computers Work* will be available.

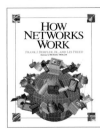
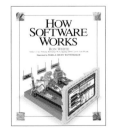
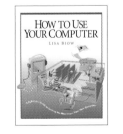
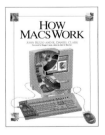

ZIFF-DAVIS
ZD
PRESS

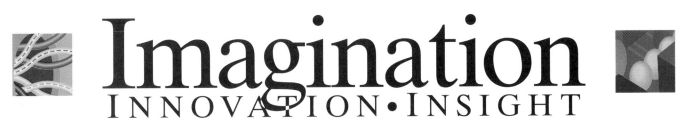
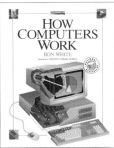
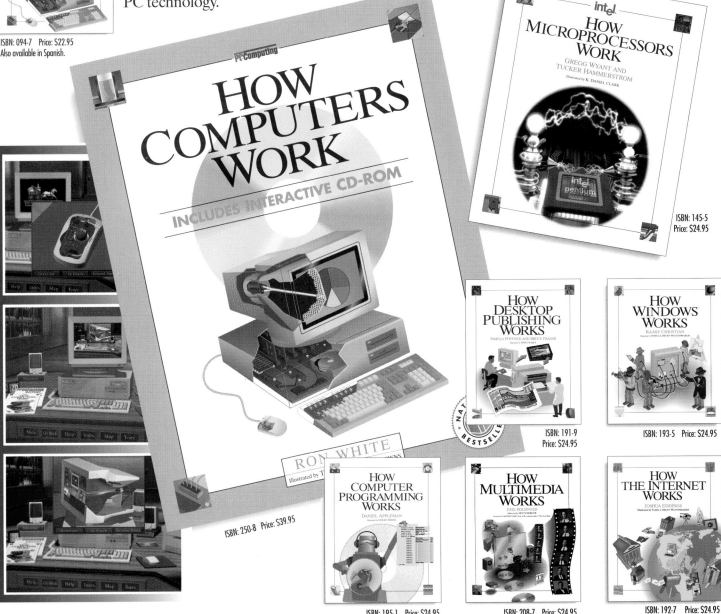

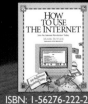
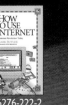
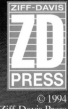